THE MYSTERY OF RISK

THE MYSTERY OF RISK

Drugs, Alcohol, Pregnancy, and the
Vulnerable Child

IRA J. CHASNOFF, MD

NTI UPSTREAM 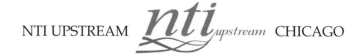 CHICAGO

NTI Upstream
180 N. Michigan Avenue, Suite 700
Chicago, Illinois 60601
Visit our website at www.ntiupstream.com

For more information about special discounts for bulk purchases or to book a live event, please contact NTI Upstream Special Sales at 1-312-423-5680.

The names of children and families in clinical cases in *The Mystery of Risk: Drugs, Alcohol, Pregnancy, and the Vunerable Child* have been changed.

Cover design by Natalie Smith
Interior design by Jennifer Fitzsimmons
Edited by Jeff Link

All photographs by NTI Upstream
Printed in the United States of America
Library of Congress Control Number 2010926911
ISBN: 978-0-9840531-5-5

To

Eva Tenberg
Junior English, Bay City High School
1964

In memorium

Ira Glick, MD
colleague, mentor, friend
1927 – 2010

To destroy abuses is not enough; habits must also be changed. The windmill has gone, but the wind is still there.

— Victor Hugo, *Les Miserables*

Prelude **Self-Portrait of a Substance-Exposed Child**

Leonard is alone. He occupies his time by pacing back and forth, crossing from one end of his cell to the other in only five strides. He's checked out some books from the library, but he can't decipher the jumble of letters and words. Ms. Rogers in second grade had tried to help him read, and one of his foster mothers — was it Mama Tess? — had even enrolled him in a Sylvan Learning Center. But before much progress could be made, he was moved again, and the next set of teachers and foster parents paid little attention to his reading skills.

Leonard's mother, painfully thin and tattooed with needle marks, had been high on crack and whiskey when he was born. The hospital records showed that Leonard was fragile and fussy and had trouble feeding. But, with no insurance to cover their stay, Leonard and his mother went home within twenty-four hours of his birth. As he grew older, Leonard's life was a haze: moving from one crack house to another, left in the care of aunts, uncles, boyfriends and strangers, some of whom paid his mother to spend time with Leonard.

Leonard remembers a younger brother, but hasn't seen him since DCFS stepped in and took custody of both boys when Leonard was five years old. Leonard was placed in an emergency foster home, but one week later the foster family called and told DCFS that someone would have to come get him. He was sexually aggressive, throwing wild tantrums that posed a danger to other children in the home. Leonard didn't fare any better with the next family, who found his frequent rages too much to handle. And so the story went. For the next seven years, Leonard went through seventeen foster homes. The placement disruptions consistently were the result of Leonard's out of control behaviors, refusal to attend school, and sexual acting out. By twelve years of age, a group home run by the Catholic Church was his last chance. During his stay over the next six years, Leonard joined a gang, began running drugs, and was arrested several times. DCFS gladly discharged Leonard from its care on his eighteenth birthday.

Homeless and alone, Leonard lived on the streets. His former DCFS caseworker kept up with him, though, and late in the first year of his emancipation, she called my office to ask if we could perform an evaluation and perhaps figure out some way to help Leonard. With Leonard's consent, we agreed to an appointment date.

Two weeks later, I was getting ready for office hours when the receptionist rang. "Leonard is here. You can come see him now." I went up to the reception area, and there, stretched the full length of one of our fake leather sofas, lay Leonard pretending to be asleep. I shook him gently and led him back to the medical examining room.

On examination, Leonard's face was a physiological map of his mother's drinking. The eyes were small and rounded, and his face was broad and flat, with a thin-lipped smile and receding chin covered in patches by a scruffy goatee. Leonard's dark skin was inked with even darker gang tattoos accompanied by a smattering of scars and bruises. He explained away some of the scars on his torso as stab wounds he had gotten in his brief bouts in lock up. But in spite of it all—his caseworker's forewarnings, his obviously low cognitive functioning, the violence that defined his past—I found Leonard's soft manner and ready laugh quite engaging.

As a last step in my part of his evaluation, I handed Leonard a piece of paper and a pencil. "Draw a person" was the only instruction I gave him. Leonard glanced at me curiously then bent forward to begin the task. I watched as his fingers gripped the pencil tightly, his eyes narrowed, and he bit his tongue with his chipped front teeth. As he drew, his free arm stubbornly guarded the page, and I was left imagining the violence and sheer gore that might emerge. But the picture was far worse than anything I had envisioned.

This was Leonard—the face, the Afro hair-do, the goatee. But the body positioning was that of an infant, with a simple message written on the front of the child's shirt. "Feed me." This was Leonard—a young man who had never had his basic needs for comfort, caring, and love met. This was Leonard—a child in a man's body, still looking for his place in the world. I lowered the piece of paper and looked Leonard in the eye. "We're going to try," was all I said.

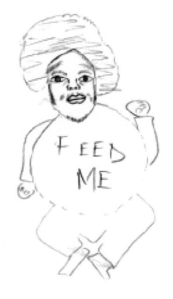

Leonard finished his two-day evaluation at our center, seen in turn by the clinical psychologist, the occupational therapist, and the education specialist. We put together a splendid intervention plan and were working hard toward a guardianship arrangement for him. But six weeks later, he was arrested once again for dealing drugs.

Leonard spends his days alone, afraid of the other prisoners who take advantage of his innocent demeanor. He has no visitors; his foster families have long forgotten him. Leonard will be almost thirty when he is released, and he likely will return to the only family who has ever accepted him—his gang brotherhood. What will happen then? The citizens and policy makers of his city, his state, and his nation will throw up their collective hands and say, "There goes another one."

Contents

PREFACE Missteps in the Dance of Attunement

There is a grace to childhood, a dance of reciprocal interactions that occurs between a child and his loving and supportive world. But just as the elegance of the finest ballet can be spoiled by a pirouette on flat feet or a floundering lift, so can a child's development suffer from missteps in the relational dance of attunement. When something goes amiss, a dance may continue to the rhythm of the music, but an underlying tension does not allow the audience — or the dancer — to relax. In the same way, when loving interactions between a parent and child are disrupted, tension and anxiety impede the child's development of emotional and relational health.

Parents shape a young child's maturation through a meaningful system of communication, providing their infant cues to guide interactions. Under ideal circumstances, the infant interprets the parent's guiding hand and responds appropriately; the parent, for her part, reads the infant's behavior and takes the next step in a well-choreographed system of interaction. This cyclical "dance of attunement" creates a balanced primary relationship that introduces the child to a trusting and trustworthy world and enables the child to take risks and grow.

Problems on either side of the equation, however, disrupt the growing relationship between parent and child. Parenting quality varies widely, with comfortable, confident parents at one end of the spectrum and anxious, depressed parents at the other. The greatest differences in parenting effectiveness lie in the ease with which the mother or father orchestrates the dialogue between parent and child; however this communication is heavily influenced by the infant's ability to interpret, interact, and respond to the parent's cues.

Infants exposed to alcohol and drugs represent a prime example of how biological damage may interfere with the child's ability to fulfill his role in the interactive dance. The pregnant woman's use of substances has a direct impact on the structure and function of the developing fetal brain and affects the child's ability to make sense of parental cues. An infant prenatally exposed to alcohol or drugs may not be as alert or engaging as a normal infant. Her parents may feel she is non-responsive, that she is "not there" for them, and as a result may fail to react sensitively to the infant's cues. To put it another way, the infant's assimilation into the family requires the development of increasingly complex skills that demonstrate the baby's growing responsiveness to parental expectations. Missteps at any point result in stumbles that damage the child's foundation for emotional and relational health.

All of this becomes more complex when the child welfare system is brought into consideration. Almost two-thirds of children identified as affected by prenatal alcohol or drug exposure are raised in out-of-home placements, and the children frequently find themselves in a foster or adoptive home unprepared to meet their needs. Foster and adoptive families who come into relationships with the children often harbor unrealistic expectations, unaware of the challenges that lie ahead. The child welfare system's lack of support to these families only further adds to the likelihood of inappropriate parenting and repeated movement of the child within the system. Disregarding permanency for the sake of expediency, rules governing the child welfare system may lead biologically vulnerable children to suffer further psychological damage in an unwittingly neglectful home. By the time the child meets his second or third set of foster parents, his heart has become like a complex work of origami, composed of intricate hidden folds that parents may find difficult if not impossible to untangle.

The purpose of this book is to examine the concept of risk from a perspective of biological vulnerability induced by prenatal exposure to alcohol and drugs and to explore how physical or emotional environmental stress can prey on that vulnerability to shape the child's future. To the observer, a child's history may be a mere record of events. But to the child, it is a life stored in memories, either known or unknown, recognized or not. Memories of early trauma or neglect can emerge at any time, driving the child's relationships, development, and achievement. While the dance of attunement may continue, if missteps are not addressed at the earliest stages of development, the cost of performance may be greater than the child can afford.

This book is written for parents, caregivers, and professionals who care for children whose development and behavior have been affected by prenatal alcohol and drug exposure, especially those children who have been ensnared in the vagaries of the child welfare system. True stories of children I have evaluated and treated during the past thirty-five years are interwoven to illustrate the importance of looking beyond the labels of risk to a path for intervention and treatment. Ultimately, the book's goal is to facilitate dialogue among parents who care for drug- and alcohol-affected children on a daily basis, professionals from a variety of disciplines who provide assessment and treatment services, and policy makers whose decisions affect the ultimate trajectory of the children's lives.

It is the book's underlying premise that labels of risk do not necessarily predict potential; risk is not destiny. Although there is no "cure" for the brain damage induced by prenatal alcohol and drug exposure, we can indeed influence a child's life for the better by redirecting him into a regulated, smooth, and mutually interactive dance with the people that matter most in his life.

— IRA J. CHASNOFF, MD

PART I
BEHAVIOR BELONGS IN THE BRAIN

1   The Long Road to Here

Morbid curiosity mixed with some bit of human sympathy has always focused professionals' and the public's attention upon errors and abnormalities of fetal development—the field of teratology. Whereas the earliest considerations of fetal maldevelopment focused on structural changes and deformities in the newly born child, for the last several decades science has come to recognize the potential for structural and functional damage that can occur in the developing fetal brain when the fetus is exposed to chemicals and other agents. The historical development of the field of teratology has brought us to our modern brain-based understanding of child development and the prenatal factors that can affect the child's behavior over the long term.

The science of teratology

Although Hippocrates and Aristotle were aware that direct injury to the embryo or increased pressure on the uterus could cause malformations, it was not until the emergence of the biological sciences in the seventeenth and eighteenth centuries that scientific explanations of fetal malformation began to develop. Most important among the explanations derived from this new way of thinking was the theory of developmental arrest, put forth by the English physician William Harvey in 1651. Harvey postulated that birth defects resulted from an arrest in an embryological process at some stage prior to its normal completion.

Experiments in teratology proliferated, until finally, in nineteen hundred, the principles of genetics were rediscovered—a full thirty-six years after Gregor Mendel first developed them. Based on Mendel's work, it was assumed that the genes that control normal development could also determine abnormal development. Fifty years later the tendency to attribute all human developmental errors to genetic deficiency had become deeply ingrained in medicine. In fact, in 1946, the *Journal of the American Medical Association* cautioned that "the offspring of alcoholics have been found defective not because of alcoholism of the parents but because the parents themselves came from a defective stock."

Modern teratology has matured over the last seventy years, stimulated by three significant events. The first of these came in 1940 when Austrian-born pediatrician Josef Warkany published studies that showed maternal dietary deficiencies in rats could cause a predictable pattern of malformations. The following year N. M. Gregg, an Australian ophthalmologist, found a high proportion of women infected with rubella (i.e., German measles) during the first three months of pregnancy gave birth to infants with malformations of multiple organs. Then, in 1961, Widukind Lenz and William McBride established the association between thalidomide consumption and the birth of severely malformed infants—eight thousand children in two years.

These events certainly illustrated the need for rigorous study of the role of environmental factors in producing congenital malformations. But the interaction of genetics and environmental factors have made it difficult to disentangle the cluster of problems arising in a family due to common genes from the cluster of problems resulting from the common environment that families share. In addition, cause-and-effect relationships are not always apparent or precise, even though scientists are regularly identifying an increasing number of damaging environmental factors. Thus, although the number of suspected causes of birth defects has increased, little is known about what really happens when normal development is disrupted, nor why this leads to such varied malformations.

One of the key problems in understanding how environmental factors can cause fetal malformations lies in the difficulty clinicians have in assessing the timing of exposure; the degree of the fetus's susceptibility to malformation varies according to when during the pregnancy the exposure occurs. There are three developmental stages most likely related to the development of a malformation:

1. The pre-differentiation period is the time from conception to implantation, about 12 to 13 days, during which the embryo is resistant to any harmful agents the mother might ingest. The embryo is resistant during this period because, prior to being implanted on the wall of the uterus, no blood or substances from the mother can reach the embryo. However, risk for death of the embryo from toxic agents ingested by the mother is greatest just before implantation.

2. In the period of early differentiation and organ development, beginning about 18 to 20 days after conception, the fetus is highly susceptible to negative influences, reaching peak sensitivity by 30 days, and ending at about 55 to 60 days. During this period there also is a high risk for fetal death from environmental toxins. Unfortunately, this is a time during which many women do not even realize they are pregnant.

3. As organ development is completed in the first trimester, susceptibility to anatomical defects diminishes greatly, but during the third trimester of pregnancy toxic agents can modify function of specific organs or induce other effects such as cell deletions or interference with tissue growth. In fact, the third trimester of pregnancy is one of the most rapid periods of brain growth throughout the human life span, and agents such as alcohol can have a tremendous adverse impact on brain growth and development during this time.

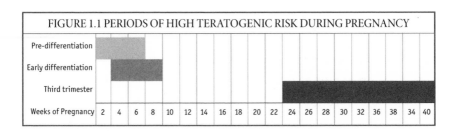

FIGURE 1.1 PERIODS OF HIGH TERATOGENIC RISK DURING PREGNANCY

Environmental influences on pregnancy and the developing fetus

As we study how environmental influences can damage pregnancy and child outcome, the first problem we run into is developing a clear definition of the fetal environment, for you cannot separate a fetus from its genetic makeup nor from the environment in which the fetus develops. For practical purposes, however, the fetal environment is the sum of all influences from outside the fetus itself.

Parental age

The age of the parents at the time of conception also has received its share of attention over the years as a factor in pregnancy outcome. The earliest congenital disorders noted to be influenced by maternal age were those due to chromosomal errors in which there were three rather than the normal two of a specific chromosome: trisomies 13, 18, or 21 (i.e., Down syndrome). There are several theories as to why older mothers produce an increased number of infants with congenital malformations:

1. Females are born with all the eggs they will have available for reproduction. The eggs accumulate damage as a result of radiation, chemicals, and infections over the woman's lifetime.

2. The placenta is more permeable to teratogenic agents in older women: harmful agents are more likely to cross the

placenta and have ready access to the developing fetus.

3. The aging uterus is less selective to defective embryos, retaining pregnancies that would have aborted when the woman was younger.
4. Fertilization of the eggs is delayed due to more infrequent coitus in older women.

No matter how old the mother, if it is a first pregnancy, there is an elevated risk for malformation. And the father is not out of the woods, either: male age at the time of conception has been directly related to the incidence of stillbirth and newborn death. Paternal age appears to be especially important in mutations that involve a single gene, probably because there are relatively few cell divisions in the female germ line but many in the male germ line; thus, the chance is greater for a gene to copy incorrectly in a man than a woman. To make things more complicated, it appears that even the age of the maternal grandfather at the time of the mother's birth has implications for the baby's health. Research has documented the age of the maternal grandfather to be a significant factor in the child's acquiring the X-linked recessive bleeding disorder hemophilia A.

Sexual and seasonal factors

In the earliest attempts to understand environmental influences on pregnancy outcome, some of the initial studies made even life's natural processes appear to be harmful. R.R. Limner, in 1969, presented an opportunity for the ultimate guilt trip in his book, *Sex and the Unborn Child*. Limner stated that sex during pregnancy deprives oxygen to the fetus at the time of maternal orgasm, resulting in abnormal development and congenital malformations in the newborn. Although this theory has been effectively dismissed by modern science, discussion of this topic is sure to induce feelings of guilt in any pregnant woman.

Still, Limmer is not alone. Studies of specific kinds of malformations have ranged from the sublime to the ridiculous.

In a 1976 New England study of congenital heart disease, the epidemiologist Kenneth Rothman and his partner Donald Fyler, a pediatric cardiologist at Harvard Medical School, documented a seasonal peak, occurring in June, in the number of newborns with transposition of the great arteries (i.e., abnormal placement of the blood vessels leading to and from the heart). Similarly, the researchers found that a higher proportion of babies were born with complex ventricular septal defect—a hole in the middle of the heart—in late summer, and abnormal positioning of the heart in autumn. Cleft lip and palate have been found to have a significantly increased prevalence from January through March; malformations of the penis have occurred most commonly in April; brain abnormalities in winter; and positional foot defects in March. Down syndrome has its peak prevalence from May through October, as do congenital hip dislocation and the sex chromosomal anomalies. There does not appear to be any absolutely safe time of year to conceive or to deliver a baby.

Maternal nutrition

The role of maternal nutrition in congenital malformation was discovered quite by accident in 1933. Pigs fed a diet deficient in vitamin A had offspring born without eyes and with cleft palates and abnormally located kidneys. Josef Warkany, known as the "father of teratology," in the early 1940s, followed up on this early information and performed animal experiments in which he fed rats a diet free of vitamin A. These rats produced newborns who were blind and had deformed eyes. He then fed the same mothers vitamin A rich diets, and the next litters had no abnormalities. Later, when Warkany restricted the vitamin riboflavin in another group of pregnant rats, the offspring were born with skeletal changes. Interestingly, these malformations were corrected if the mothers were fed riboflavin on days 13 and 14 of gestation—the period of bone development in rats.

Around the same time, World War II presented an opportunity to study the effects of more generalized maternal undernutrition. Using time before the war and after the war as controls, Clement Smith, a pioneer in the field of neonatology, studied the effect of a three- to four-month Nazi-imposed food blockade of Holland. During this time, Holland's urban population showed a markedly decreased intake of calories and vitamins. Smith found 50% of the country's women stopped having periods. Nine months after the blockade, there was one-third the usual number of births. For pregnancies already underway—in which mothers were deprived of food during the last three months of gestation—there was a very high rate of babies born below normal birth weight. However, malnutrition did not produce low birth weight infants if the malnutrition occurred in the first six months of gestation. Nor was any relation found between maternal nutrition and rates of abortion, stillbirth, or newborn death. The World Health Organization, on the other hand, has studied malnourished women worldwide and found an increased rate of early abortions and stillbirths, though no conclusive evidence of malformations.

Radiation exposure

World War II provided a chance to study several other teratogenic agents, not the least of which was the atomic bomb. As early as 1911, radiation exposure during gestation had been shown to cause leukemia in the child; and in 1929 there were several reports of children being born with small brains, skull and spinal cord defects, cleft palate, and club foot to women who received large doses of pelvic radiation by X-ray or radium.

For those fetuses exposed to the atomic bombs in Japan—if they were exposed at fewer than 18 weeks gestation, with a dose below 20 rads—8% were born with a small brain (i.e., microcephaly). The rate of microcephaly increased proportionately with increased dose of radiation, so that in utero exposure at fewer than 18 weeks, with 150 rads, produced microcephaly in 59% of the newborns. In studies with pregnant rats, exposure to successive doses of radiation at 10 days gestation demonstrated a very clear dose response curve, with heavy doses resulting in fetal death within 24 hours of exposure. At the same time, escalating damage has been found when rats are irradiated at a standardized dosage at different gestational ages. Thus, it continues to be unclear whether the patterns of malformation due to radiation exposure are governed chiefly by the timing of injury or by the intensity of radiation.

Pollution

In recent decades, as environmental pollution has become a defining political issue, scientists have turned their attention to the effects this pollution may have on the fetus. In studies of metropolitan areas of the United States, those areas with the most air pollution have the lowest birth rates and the highest prevalence of congenital malformation and newborn death. However, these data have not been consistently verified, and additional factors, such as nutrition and socioeconomics, make it very difficult to understand the impact of pollution on pregnancy outcome. One last bit of potential bad news for city dwellers: pregnant rats exposed to noise stress of 74 to 94 decibels, for 2.5 hours every day, produced offspring with altered skeletal systems and poor bone formation.

Maternal diabetes

As we move from external to internal factors, we find that the metabolic environment the fetus inhabits is altered by a broad spectrum of maternal diseases, not the least of which is diabetes. The association of maternal diabetes with fetal malformations has been well documented, but controversy persists as to the magnitude of the risk to the fetus. Prevalence of congenital abnormalities among diabetic women is reported to range from 0% to 20%. Difficulty in making an exact determination lies in the various criteria for recognizing diabetes. In one study that reviewed the outcomes of 7,101 fetuses and infants of diabetic mothers, 340, or about 5%, were malformed as opposed to the 2% malformation prevalence in the general population. Other studies have found the rate of congenital malformations in infants of diabetic mothers three times more than the rate of malformation for non-diabetic mothers, and the death rate six times higher. The frequency and severity of the malformations were higher in infants of mothers with more severe vascular complications related to their diabetes.

When considering women who are not diagnosed with diabetes but simply have an abnormal glucose tolerance test during pregnancy, there is no increase in infant mortality or in rates of malformation. However, in an attempt to investigate the issue from a different vantage, one researcher identified two distinct populations of babies—one population with congenital malformation and the other without malformations—and administered glucose tolerance tests to their mothers. There was a significantly increased prevalence of abnormal glucose tolerance tests in the mothers with malformed infants. Thus, it seems the jury is still out as to whether a pre-diabetic condition produces risk for malformations in the child.

Maternal substance abuse

It was not until after the thalidomide disaster that scientists turned their attention to fetal damage medications and other drugs might cause; foremost among these was tobacco. Several studies have documented a significant increase in rates of low birth weight, premature birth, and infant death in babies born to mothers who smoke. There also is an increased incidence of spontaneous abortions among smokers, which is directly related to the number of cigarettes smoked per day. In one study, children born to smoking mothers have been found, at seven years of age, to be shorter and to suffer an increased prevalence of educational challenges and difficulties, including attention-deficit/hyperactivity disorder (ADHD). This remains true even when several control factors are held constant, including social class, number of pregnancies, and maternal age and height. This study also found that infant death was lowest for non-smoking mothers and highest for mothers who smoked more than four cigarettes per day. The number of cigarettes smoked after four months of pregnancy was the most significant predictor in the occurrence of newborn deaths and low birth weight, regardless of smoking history prior to pregnancy or in early pregnancy.

The danger of drinking alcohol during pregnancy has been recognized since Biblical times. Aristotle wrote of the harm done to the unborn child by alcohol use in pregnancy, and wood etchings from the seventeen hundreds depicting the scourge of the gin epidemic in England portray children with facial features characteristic of fetal alcohol syndrome (FAS). Yet modern medicine has been slow to identify the risks of alcohol use during pregnancy. Eventually, in France, in 1967, the physician Philip Lemoine and his colleagues described fetal alcohol syndrome and the associated malformations and mental retardation that occur in the exposed child. Around the same time, Ken Jones and David Smith, pediatricians at the University of Washington School of Medicine, recognized eight children enrolled in their Failure to Thrive clinic whose mothers had drunk alcohol during pregnancy and who had characteristics similar to those described by the French. In spite of the publication of this information in the British medical journal *Lancet*, controversy surrounded these findings for years. In the United States, known for widespread use of alcohol as a social stimulant, many were reluctant to recognize the danger of drinking during pregnancy.

Behavioral teratology

As devastating as it has been in other ways, one rare benefit of the crack epidemic was that it opened the field of behavioral teratology to broader inquiry. Scientists and the public began to realize that children's exposure to substances ingested by a pregnant woman could affect the child's brain function without causing obvious physical disfigurement or malformation. As physicians, we had before us a population of children who "looked normal" but had significant behavioral and developmental problems, some of which were quite subtle but nonetheless affected day-to-day functioning.

Since then, the body of literature exploring behavioral teratology as affected by prenatal alcohol and drug exposure has grown rapidly, especially with the advent of sophisticated imaging techniques such as MRIs and CAT scans. It is clear that children exposed prenatally to maternal substances of abuse are at risk across multiple areas of function. However, studies of the exact impact of alcohol and drug use in pregnancy on child behavior outcome are hampered by a number of factors:

1. Most investigations are retrospective and evaluate children only by assessing past experiences and exposures. Though prospective studies are feasible, interpretation is complicated by the nature, timing, and dose of the suspected drug.
2. Investigation of alcohol and other drugs a woman takes during pregnancy involves two biological systems, both the placenta and the mother's metabolic processes modifying the agent before it reaches the fetus. That makes it difficult to locate the origin of biological damage.
3. Information regarding timing of the fetus's exposure to alcohol or other drugs is unreliable, relying on the mother's recall of her use patterns.
4. Classic randomization methods are impossible due to ethical concerns. How could we ever say to a group of pregnant women, "OK, you take cocaine, and you don't. You drink alcohol, and you don't."

As gradual as research has been in defining the specific effects of prenatal exposure on child outcome, attempts to develop appropriate intervention strategies for children have gone even more slowly. One great deterrent to progress is that even the most sophisticated of modern studies continue to be conducted from a deficit perspective. Research studies of children affected by prenatal exposure to alcohol and illicit drugs tend to determine, first, how exposed children differ from the rest of us, only to define those differences as the cause of any problems we find in the children. Programs are set up to correct the differences. However, this kind of deficit approach allows us to ignore factors that are not under the lens of investigation such as poverty, homelessness, and poor access to health care. A narrow focus on "differences" also provides government agencies with an excuse to neglect serious attempts toward more long-term, comprehensive solutions.

The British researcher David J. P. Barker and his partner Clive Osmond, a statistician, found themselves thrust into the midst of this controversy with their investigation of how low birth weight and infant growth influence the occurrence of major illness in adulthood. Termed the "Barker hypothesis," these researchers found that poor nutrition during prenatal and early infant life was related to later heart disease. A storm of debate followed the initial publication of their thesis, but before long Barker and Osmond had corroboration. Using low birth weight as a marker of risk, researchers began to find a consistent pattern: poor growth in the womb was associated with increased risk for coronary heart disease, hypertension, type 2 diabetes, and stroke in the adult. Nonetheless, "correlation is not causation," and clinical studies to explain the epidemiologic patterns continue amid dissension.

Besides illustrating difficulties inherent in trying to understand the impact of prenatal drug and alcohol exposure on the child, controversy in the wake of the Barker hypothesis shines a light on the media's role in conflating the process of scientific discovery. Indeed, you cannot have a meaningful discussion of the effects of prenatal exposure to illicit drugs, especially cocaine, without acknowledging the role the media have played in coloring the public and professional view of these children. When the first article regarding cocaine use in pregnancy was published in the

New England Journal of Medicine in 1985, there was an immediate reaction from the media. Although the scientific report addressed only the impact of cocaine on pregnancy and the newborn, the media jumped way ahead of research, concocting grim hypotheses about the long-term impact of exposure. Many researchers, this one included, saw articles in the popular press that headed into untoward directions, leaving many of us to wonder where communication of the scientific evidence had gone wrong.

This media phenomenon occurred, of course, within the context and times of the "war on drugs." Although initiated by Richard Nixon in 1971 during the waning days of his administration, the federal effort to address drug abuse did not really gather steam until President Reagan declared his intent to wipe out the scourge of drug abuse in the nation, signing the Anti-Drug Abuse Act of 1986. The act appropriated $1.7 billion to fight the drug crisis, including $200 million for drug education, $241 million for drug treatment, and $97 million to build prisons. The aspect of the bill with the most far-reaching implications was the creation of a mandatory minimum penalty for drug offenses. From the beginning, the war on drugs was an ill-conceived policy, off track in its attempt to distinguish the "bad" drugs from the "good" drugs. Cocaine, heroin, PCP were bad drugs—everyone agreed to that. Tobacco and alcohol were viewed as good drugs—the lobbyists for the alcohol and tobacco industries made sure to protect their investments. And no one quite knew what to do with marijuana.

From a social perspective, cocaine and heroin were identified as drugs of choice for inner-city blacks. Tobacco and alcohol were the drugs preferred by the white middle class. Most assuredly, if alcohol and tobacco had been included in the federal effort, the term "war on drugs" never would have been used—waging war against the white middle class, from the administration's perspective, was to risk political suicide. Consequently, the war on drugs leveled stiffer criminal penalties at drugs viewed as more prevalent within the African-American community. Discrepant sentencing laws made crack use a greater offense than powder cocaine use — possessing fifty grams of crack, compared with five thousand grams of powder cocaine, earned a ten-year minimum sentence — though scientific evidence showed crack and cocaine were physiologically identical substances. Newspapers filled their pages with images of black inner city youth and adults being hauled off to prison for their crack and heroin use. Rarely did newspapers show the pictures of white youth who were using cocaine in record numbers.

Set against this background, our research team published a follow-up article in 1992, which showed that prenatal cocaine exposure did not have any direct effect on the status of the child's cognitive development at two and three years old. We followed this with another study documenting that, although behavior of cocaine-exposed children suffered from direct exposure to cocaine, the environment in which the child was raised had a stronger impact than cocaine exposure on long-term cognitive outcome. After the publication of these articles, there was an abrupt turn-around in the media. Now headlines announced that there was no real danger from crack or cocaine use in pregnancy. Moving from one extreme to the other, the media again got it wrong. Early intervention programs, maternal drug treatment programs, policies to protect children — all were being swept aside on the justification of the media's rush to judgment.

To this day, many professionals continue to oppose the idea that alcohol or illicit drugs have any significant impact on child development and behavior. However, from a biological perspective, numerous scientific studies make it clear that prenatal exposure to alcohol, tobacco or illicit drugs has a teratogenic effect on the developing fetal brain, resulting in structural and functional changes. These changes can affect behavior and development and make the growing child more vulnerable to damage from environmental factors such as abuse, neglect, and exposure to violence. Neither nature nor nurture alone guides the trajectory of child development. Instead it is an integration of biological and environmental factors that have direct impact on the developing fetal brain and the brain of the young child.

Bruce Perry, a child's mental health specialist and Senior Fellow of the Child Trauma Academy in Houston, Texas, expresses this integration of nature and nurture elegantly when he writes of a neurosequential model of development. In this model, Perry postulates that children who grow up in chaotic and threatening environments do not have the fundamental developmental experiences that support healthy maturation of their neurological systems. A traumatized child's cognitive, behavioral, and emotional functioning stall at the developmental point at which trauma is suffered. If we locate trauma inside the birth environment, this harkens back to Harvey's theory of developmental arrest. It seems we have come full circle. Now, with modern brain imaging techniques, we are embarking on a whole new era of research and clinical services, armed with the knowledge that behavior belongs in the brain.

2 Alcohol, Aristotle, and Swiss Cheese

Foolish, drunken, or harebrain women most often bring forth children like unto themselves.

— Aristotle, *Problemata*

At the age of six, Jonny looks like a rounded, well-hued block of marble. He wears his hair cropped closely to the scalp and has the hard, determined look of a soldier. "Rages," his adoptive father says in his country drawl. "Jonny shows rages." During his outbursts, which occur daily and occasionally last over an hour, Jonny swears, hits, kicks, spits, and destroys property. Some of his rages require him to be physically restrained.

Jonny's prenatal and early childhood experiences are practically unimaginable. In the fog of her alcoholism, his biological mother attempted to abort him with a wire coat hanger. He still has the scars on his abdomen to prove it. He was delivered into his mother's toilet three months before the due date, weighing one pound fifteen ounces. As soon as he was born, his mother wrapped him in a plastic bag and threw him into a garbage can outside her apartment. A little later, she saw the bag moving and took the child to the hospital. He spent the first several months of his life in the neonatal intensive care unit and was sent to his adoptive parents' home immediately upon release. He sometimes still asks where his mother is.

Jonny is a busy boy; his adoptive parents describe him as a whirlwind. He often can be seen in our clinic hurdling the couches in the waiting room or randomly banging into the walls. With an IQ in the mid- to high-70s, it is difficult to find the right educational environment to suit his needs. Jonny's intellectual deficits often are manifest in poor comprehension—and a porous memory one of his teachers likens to Swiss cheese: "One day he'll seem to have mastery in a certain academic area and then the next day it's totally gone, but then might be back the following day. It's kind of like some days, he knows how to pull out the information and other days he doesn't. There are holes where things fall in and out. It's like Swiss cheese."

Over the last several decades, progress has been slow in determining how many children in this country are affected by prenatal exposure to alcohol. A combination of legal, social, and attitudinal barriers has restrained communication on every level, starting with the health care provider and patient. Physicians rarely ask a pregnant woman about her alcohol intake, and fetal alcohol syndrome (FAS) remains the most common cause of diagnosable mental retardation in the United States as well as one of the leading causes of behavioral problems in children.

The prevalence of FAS is estimated to range from 0.2 to 2 cases per 1,000 live births, depending on ethnic, cultural, and regional factors. Given the approximately 4 million births per year in the United States, there are up to 6,000 children born each year with FAS. But the problem is even worse than these statistics suggest. A recent study of 4,800 women from a wide range of social and economic classes found that 22% of the women had used alcohol in early pregnancy and 11% continued drinking even though they knew they were pregnant. Thus, about 1 million children across the United States may be exposed prenatally to alcohol each year. These children can suffer from a broad range of difficulties that, while often quite subtle, can compromise the children's long-term health, behavior, development, and academic achievement.

Criteria for diagnosis

Fetal alcohol syndrome is the original name given to a cluster of physical and mental defects present from birth that is the direct result of a woman's drinking alcoholic beverages while pregnant. Infants with FAS have signs in three categories: (1) growth deficiencies (2) central nervous system impairment and (3) facial dysmorphology.

The mother's confirmed use of alcohol is not necessary to make a diagnosis of FAS if the child meets criteria in all three categories. However, to ensure accuracy and completeness in the child's medical records, physicians should note when the diagnosis is based solely on these physical and developmental parameters and without confirmation of the mother's drinking.

As we begin this discussion, it is important to realize that the impact of prenatal alcohol exposure is not determined only by the cumulative "dose" of alcohol to which the child was exposed. Many reports demonstrate that the mother's binge drinking, with high peak blood alcohol levels, is actually more dangerous than chronic drinking. A recent report regarding adolescents noted, in addition, that as little as one drink per week during pregnancy has a significant detrimental impact on the child's weight at fourteen years of age. Animal studies have demonstrated that even small amounts of alcohol affect neurodevelopment in adolescence.

Growth deficiencies

In the United States, the average birth weight of babies born at full term (38 to 42 weeks gestation) is 7 pounds 8 ounces, with a normal range down to 5 pounds 8 ounces. Babies born to mothers who use alcohol have an average birth weight of around 6 pounds and are more likely than babies born to mothers who abstained to weigh less than 5 pounds 8 ounces. As children with fetal alcohol syndrome grow older, they tend to continue to be small for their age—that is, short and underweight. To meet the FAS diagnostic guidelines set for growth criteria, a child must have either reduced weight *or* height (at or below 10th percentile on standard growth charts) at birth *or* at any point in time after birth.

Changes in facial features

Facial features associated with prenatal alcohol exposure are consistent with overall flattening of the middle portion of the face. As a result, children with FAS exhibit:

- Epicanthal folds (extra skin folds coming down around the inner angle of the eye)
- Short palpebral fissures (small eye openings)
- A flattened elongated philtrum (no groove or crease running from the bottom of the nose to the top of the lip)
- Thin upper lip
- Small mouth with high arched palate (roof of the mouth)
- Small teeth with poor enamel coating
- Low set ears

These changes can vary in severity, but usually persist over the life of the child. Most people will not recognize any differences when they see the child, but physicians and other practitioners with experience in working with children prenatally exposed to alcohol will be able to detect the changes.

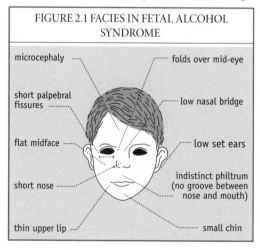

FIGURE 2.1 FACIES IN FETAL ALCOHOL SYNDROME

microcephaly

folds over mid-eye

short palpebral fissures

low nasal bridge

flat midface

low set ears

short nose

indistinct philtrum (no groove between nose and mouth)

thin upper lip

small chin

A problem arises when clinicians rely too heavily on changes in facial structure to recognize the child affected by prenatal alcohol exposure. In animal studies, pregnant rats given alcohol on days 7 or 8 after conception had newborns with facial features typical of FAS. However, giving the pregnant rats alcohol on days 1 through 6, or on day 9 or any time beyond, did not affect the facial features in any way. Thus, there appears to be a very narrow window of alcohol exposure that can affect children's facial features.

Children with fetal alcohol syndrome also may have a variety of malformations of major organs, especially the heart, kidneys, eyes, and ears. Children with prenatal alcohol exposure frequently have vision problems; many have an eye that turns inward (i.e., esotropia, or a "lazy eye"). In addition, the children can have a predisposition to ear infections and a high rate of partial or complete hearing loss (i.e., eighth nerve deafness), so a thorough hearing exam is recommended in the first year of life and should be repeated annually based on the child's speech and language development.

Central nervous system impairment

Problems in the central nervous system can become manifest through structural, neurological, or functional changes. Structurally, a small head circumference (at or below 10th percentile) at birth or at any time thereafter indicates poor brain growth. For example, the average head size of term infants at birth is 35 centimeters, while the head size of a baby with FAS often is less than 33 centimeters. Neurological damage can be manifest as seizures, problems in coordination, difficulty with motor control, or a number of "soft" neurological deficits. Functionally, the average IQ in children with FAS is about 68, as compared to the general population in which the average IQ is 100. Alcohol-exposed children, with or without the characteristic facial features or growth retardation, have consistently lower IQ scores than non-exposed children. Importantly, even alcohol-exposed children with a "normal IQ" demonstrate difficulty with behavioral regulation, impulsivity, social deficits, and poor judgment, causing problems in day-to-day management in the classroom and home.

In fact, children with FAS exhibit a wide range of functional difficulties much more common than mental retardation; these difficulties include learning disabilities, poor school performance, diminished executive functioning (e.g., organization of tasks, understanding cause and effect, following several steps of directions), clumsiness, poor balance, and problems with writing or drawing. Behaviorally, many of the children have a short attention span, and often are described as impulsive and hyperactive.

From a brain structure perspective, prenatal alcohol exposure not only can cause the child to have a small brain overall but also can stunt the growth of individual parts of the brain. This damaged growth may be present regardless of the child's facial features. Problems with the formation and development of different parts of the brain can result in a wide range of behavioral and learning deficits. Many children with prenatal alcohol exposure have trouble moving information between different brain regions; they cannot effectively use information to self-direct their behavior or to think in the abstract. They may have trouble learning new information and recording it in the brain—and then have even more difficulty retrieving the information they've already learned. Like Jonny, a child may learn his multiplication tables one day, but forget them the next.

Other parts of the brain also can be affected, impairing the child's ability to coordinate planned motor movements and resulting in impulsive movement and clumsiness. Reduction in the size of the cerebellum in the back part of the brain, for example, produces difficulties with balance and arousal and may be a source of sleep problems. Again, it is important to remember that such problems occur not only in children with the abnormal facial features associated with full expression of FAS, but also in alcohol-exposed children who "look normal."

Another way alcohol can affect brain functioning is by disrupting sugar metabolism in the brain, which may lead to a clinical pattern of distractibility and impulsiveness. Worse, many alcohol-exposed children are simultaneously exposed to their mother's gestational use of tobacco, cocaine, methamphetamine, heroin, marijuana, and other drugs. These substances affect the dopamine, serotonin, and norepinephrine systems in the fetal brain, causing changes in the composition of chemicals that control behavior, thought, emotions, and movement. Thus, the exposed child has trouble responding appropriately to the world around him and looks "out of sync" in the classroom and at home. The difficulty in evaluating and diagnosing children with prenatal alcohol exposure often lies in separating the effects of the alcohol exposure from the effects of the tobacco or other drugs to which the child was exposed.

Brain structure and function: Deficits in information processing

The behavioral, emotional, and learning difficulties of children with prenatal alcohol exposure can be best understood as a deficit in processing information. More specifically, children have difficulty recording information (bringing it into the brain); interpreting information; storing information in memory for later use; and using information to guide actions, behavior, emotions, language, and movement. The normal magnetic resonance imaging (MRI) shown in Figure 2.2 demonstrates some key brain structures and areas affected by drug and alcohol exposure. The cerebral cortex is the outer shell of the brain; the prefrontal cortex is a component of the overall cortex, the area that contains dopamine and serves as the regulatory center of the brain; the corpus callosum is a part of the limbic system, located in the exact midline of the brain.

Damage from drinking in the first trimester — that is, the first three months of pregnancy — mainly occurs in the midline

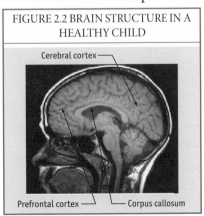

FIGURE 2.2 BRAIN STRUCTURE IN A HEALTHY CHILD

Cerebral cortex

Prefrontal cortex — Corpus callosum

structures of the brain, where the limbic system is located. The limbic system guides information processing: the way we bring information into the brain and use it to manage our behaviors, emotions, and thoughts. As seen in Figure 2.3, data retrieved from our senses enters the brain through different pathways. Visual information enters through the back portion of the brain, a region known as the occipital lobe. Touch, taste, and smell enter through the parietal lobe, located in the upper, posterior half of the brain. Auditory information enters through the ear, and the eighth cranial nerve carries the information from the ear to the inner midline section of the brain.

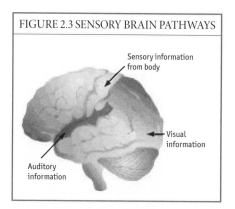

FIGURE 2.3 SENSORY BRAIN PATHWAYS

Sensory information from body

Visual information

Auditory information

A primary job of the brain is to bring these disparate bits of sensory input together and conduct the information to the prefrontal cortex in the front of the brain. There, dopamine, a key neurotransmitter, is fired off at intervals to guide the individual in using and responding appropriately to the information via motor activity, behavior, emotion, speech and language. In other words, by regulating the amount and frequency of dopamine release, the individual is able to use information *from* the environment to manage a response *to* the environment.

Alcohol's damage to the limbic system is what produces many of the functional difficulties we see in children exposed prenatally to alcohol. For example, the hippocampus, situated in the posterior aspect of the limbic system, plays a role in consolidating new memories and applying information in novel situations. If the hippocampus is damaged, the child has difficulty transferring neurologically generated maps of information and experience to long-term memory storehouses in the temporal lobes. The child may know, cognitively, not to run out into a particular street in front of his house, but cannot retrieve that knowledge when approaching a different street. As a result, he runs out into the street, appearing to be "impulsive" or "hyperactive."

Other alcohol-induced structural changes in the brain can occur in the corpus callosum, the portion of the brain that permits the two major halves to share information. When compared to the normal MRI seen previously (Figure 2.2), the corpus callosum in the MRI of the child with FAS (Figure 2.4) is narrower at its posterior segment. This structural thinning effect disrupts communication within the brain so that certain types of information can never reach consciousness. For example, an alcohol-exposed child may be able to recite the rules for good behavior in the school lunchroom, but be unable to regulate his behavior in accordance with those rules. As a result, he is described as disobedient or labeled with a diagnosis of oppositional defiant disorder (ODD): "He knows what he's supposed to do," exclaims his teacher. "He just won't do it!" Although a child with FAS may meet diagnostic criteria for oppositional defiant disorder, diagnostic and therapeutic approaches must consider the nature of the structural brain defects that are producing the behavior before such a determination is made. We are asking clinicians and parents to look beyond the behavior they see to identify the root cause of that behavior.

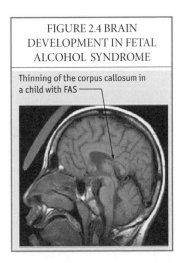

FIGURE 2.4 BRAIN DEVELOPMENT IN FETAL ALCOHOL SYNDROME

Thinning of the corpus callosum in a child with FAS

Finally, the thalamus (also part of the limbic system) receives input from all over the body and sends it to the cerebral cortex, the area of the brain responsible for cognition and learning. The thalamus also helps organize behavior related to survival: fighting, feeding, and fleeing. That is why children with FAS often get a panicked look in their eyes when faced with a sudden change or threat, or overloaded with information. When parents describe the children as being "stubborn," they are recognizing, perhaps, that the child diagnosed with FAS does not learn from experience in the same way other children do. This is not willful behavior on the part of the child; rather, the connections between past instructions or experience and current behavior just don't exist.

Alcohol use in the third trimester—the final three months of pregnancy—causes damage to the cerebral cortex, the outer shell of the brain. In the normal MRI shown previously (Figure 2.2), the cortex is folded in upon itself, forming the *gyri* and *sulci*, or valleys and ridges, in the brain. This folding occurs in the third trimester, producing increased brain surface area. In general, the more brain surface present in the cortex, the higher the level of cognitive functioning.

When a woman uses alcohol during the third trimester, however, brain cell migration is disrupted, interfering with the development of the gyri and sulci and significantly reducing brain surface area. As seen in Figure 2.5, also a MRI of a child with FAS, the brain is small in circumference, there are very few folds in the cortex of the brain, and the surface of the brain is quite flat (known as lisencephaly). These changes may be among the major factors producing the mental retardation seen in many children with FAS.

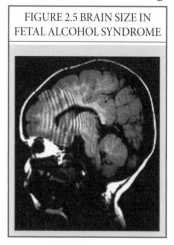

FIGURE 2.5 BRAIN SIZE IN FETAL ALCOHOL SYNDROME

Terminology

For the past thirty years, if a woman drank alcohol during pregnancy and gave birth to a child who showed partial or no apparent expression of physical features characteristic of alcohol exposure, her child was said to have fetal alcohol effects (FAE). These children may have had minimal to moderate facial changes or no changes at all, but usually they had some problems with intellectual, behavioral, or emotional development. These difficulties were known to have an impact on learning and long-term development, though just how extensively FAE affected the child was less clear.

More recently, research has demonstrated that children with FAE may have significant structural and functional changes in the brain, even though they lack overt physical manifestation of the alcohol exposure. Currently, the preferred terminology for children who have been exposed to alcohol but who do not meet criteria in all three diagnostic categories is alcohol-related neurodevelopmental disorder (ARND) or alcohol-related birth defects (ARBD). In April 2004, a group of federal agencies developed a consensus definition of fetal alcohol spectrum disorders (FASD):

> [A]n umbrella term describing the range of effects that can occur in an individual whose mother drank during pregnancy. These effects may include physical, mental, behavioral, and/or learning disabilities with possible lifelong implications.   (Bertrand et al., 2004)

Diagnostic terminology in daily use mainly focuses on FAS or ARND, both of which fall within the larger continuum of effects seen in children with FASD. FASD is not meant to serve as a diagnostic term, but rather a unifying one to help us appreciate the many ways in which prenatal alcohol exposure can become manifest in the affected individual. For our purposes, we will use the term "FASD" when the information applies to all alcohol-exposed children, including those with a diagnosis of FAS, ARND, or ARBD. When the information specifically refers to children with FAS or ARND, we will use those terms.

Diagnostic dilemmas

If diagnosis of alcohol-affected children were as easy as the terminology implies, we could move on from this discussion to other more important topics. But the truth is there is great controversy as to how and when to diagnose children whose mothers drank alcohol during pregnancy. The key barrier to diagnosis is the lack of information regarding maternal alcohol use during pregnancy. Recent studies in general populations of pregnant women report that anywhere from 16% to 35% of the women have drunk some amount of alcohol during gestation, with the highest risk population frequently comprising middle class, well-educated women. However, prenatal care providers often are reluctant to address their patients' drinking, and as a result alcohol use continues to lead to FASD—one of the most commonly missed complications of pregnancy.

Another difficulty in diagnosis relates to the lack of physical sequelae among the majority of alcohol-exposed children. Through the history of work with FAS, facial changes have been recognized as an essential component of diagnosis. In 2001, the researchers Susan Astley and Sterling Clarren evaluated the correlation of facial changes with brain dysfunction in a population of alcohol-exposed children. The authors found that children with more severe facial changes demonstrated more severely impaired levels of cognitive, neuropsychological, and visual motor functioning. More recently, Astley emphasized the importance of the specificity of facial criteria in concluding a child has FAS. However, at the same time, new research is demonstrating the primary role growth status (height and weight) has in recognizing children at risk from prenatal alcohol exposure. In a recent study at Children's Research Triangle, among 78 foster and adopted children with a confirmed history of prenatal alcohol exposure, the children's current growth patterns, as opposed to facial changes, provided the strongest correlations with poor neurodevelopmental functioning. In this same study, by restricting the diagnosis of FAS to children with growth below the 3rd percentile rather than the 10th percentile for chronological age, we were able to demonstrate neurodevelopmental differences between children with FAS vs. ARND.

The clarification of these diagnostic issues is important for all those who care for children, especially pediatricians whose role is to recognize, early, those children who may be at risk from prenatal exposure to alcohol and foster and adoptive parents who must advocate for the child to ensure access to early intervention programs. Without a diagnosis of alcohol-related risk, many children will not be deemed eligible for early intervention and school-based treatment programs, nor will insurance companies pay for related health care interventions. Parents and caregivers thus find themselves in a position of advocating for children not deemed "sick enough" to receive services.

In October 2005, the Centers for Disease Control and Prevention (CDC) published guidelines for the identification and referral of persons with fetal alcohol syndrome. The underlying goal of their report was to clarify the diagnosis of FAS, so as to enhance practicing clinicians' ability to recognize and refer patients who may have been negatively affected by prenatal alcohol exposure. However, for practicing clinicians, the CDC's guidelines contain many confusing features. The recommendation that substantial prenatal alcohol use must be confirmed runs counter to published data that document the impact of relatively small amounts of alcohol use in pregnancy. Further, any thresholds for safe use have not been empirically validated, and as the authors of the CDC article acknowledge, it is extremely difficult to confirm prenatal alcohol use because denial, minimization, and inaccurate memories in birth parents are common.

In addition, the collection of some of the data recommended in the CDC guidelines lies outside the practice of a general pediatric office. While it is relatively straightforward to evaluate more evident changes in the midface (nose, lip), it is extremely difficult to measure palpebral fissure size (i.e., size of the eye) without special equipment and facilities. From a practical perspective, many of the recommendations are overly broad: referring all children proposed in the CDC's 2005 published guidelines—those with alcoholic parents, history of abuse or neglect, involvement with the child welfare system, or history of foster or adoptive placements — simply is not viable. Presently, further research is necessary to develop a more practical and clinically appropriate approach for the recognition and diagnosis of the spectrum of alcohol-related sequelae in children. Most importantly, eligibility criteria for the various federal- and state-funded treatment programs must be expanded to include all children at risk from prenatal alcohol exposure.

3 Toddlers, Toxins, and Smearing Feces

Five-month-old Andrew lay propped in his foster mother's lap, vacant eyes lost in an oddly shaped face, his head always tilted to the right. The cooing and funny faces, which almost always elicit smiles from babies his age, went unnoticed. The reaching and grabbing expected when brightly colored toys were dangled in front of him were inhibited by the limited use of his arms. His foster parents, who had been caring for Andrew since his mother, a cocaine addict, had given birth to him, described Andrew as passive and lethargic. He trembled at the slightest stimulation. He spent most of his day sleeping, and when he was not being entertained, he would quickly drift off. His wandering gaze and expressionless face made you wonder how much of him was really there. But in spite of it all, his new family was falling in love with the sweet, good-natured baby they had taken into their care.

Andrew's development lagged, as he grew older. He fell farther and farther behind, functioning at the level of a fifteen-month-old when he was two-and-a-half years old. Added to the developmental delays, Andrew was having upwards of twenty temper tantrums a day, could not sleep for more than three hours at a time, and had a nightly ritual of banging his head and screaming. He had changed from a listless child to one who was never still. He whirled around a room—expending the most energy moving toys in and out of a garbage can, grunting and pointing in attempts at communication, and most disturbingly for his parents, smearing his feces on any available wall.

When it comes to drug use, one of the major differences between men and women is that women addicts are polydrug users while men typically use only one drug. This places children whose mothers use substances during pregnancy at high risk for exposure to multiple drugs. Indeed, it is not uncommon to find a child who has been simultaneously exposed to cocaine, methamphetamine, tobacco, alcohol, and marijuana, with multiple areas of the fetal brain affected. So while an alcohol-exposed child may have changes in the limbic system due to the effect of the mother's alcohol consumption, prenatal exposure to cocaine, methamphetamine, tobacco, marijuana, and other illicit substances adds to the problem by causing changes in the prefrontal cortex.

How drugs work

To understand how drugs act on the nervous system, one first must understand how the nervous system works. If you want your fingers to wiggle, you send an electrical message from your brain to your fingers to wiggle. There is not one long nerve leading from the brain to the fingers, but a series of nerves through which the electrical stimulus must travel. In order to move from one nerve to the next, the stimulus is picked up at the end of the first nerve by a set of neurotransmitters and carried across the nerve gap to the next nerve. After the neurotransmitters release the electrical stimulus so that it can continue down the nerve pathway, they circulate back to the first nerve ending, a process known as "reuptake." Thus, there is a steady supply of neurotransmitters always at the ready to serve as the regulatory center of the brain.

Almost all drugs of abuse, from tobacco to cocaine, from methamphetamine to marijuana, act on the neurotransmitter system in the brain. One of the key neurotransmitters is dopamine, especially important in the context of drug use because dopamine serves as the pleasure center of the brain. Drug addicts use drugs because the drugs cause an increase in the amount of dopamine available at nerve endings. This elevated level of dopamine is the "high" achieved by drug use.

Cocaine and methamphetamine serve as good counterpoints for explaining how drug use affects the dopamine receptor system. In simplest terms, cocaine blocks dopamine reuptake, while methamphetamine causes an excess release of dopamine in the brain. In both cases, the drugs produce a "high" by increasing the amount of dopamine available at the nerve ends and thereby increasing the excitation of the nerves. However, over a period of chronic exposure to cocaine or methamphetamine (or other drugs of abuse, including nicotine) a dampening effect may occur, resulting in the depletion of dopamine receptors. This may make a person feel off task, irritable, and confused, and cause difficulties in concentration. The only way to overcome these feelings is to replenish the dopamine levels at the nerve endings by taking more drugs.

On the neurological level, this dopamine cycle explains the process of addiction. Drug addicts begin using drugs to feel good, but they keep using drugs so they won't feel bad. With progressively less dopamine in the prefrontal cortex, it takes an ever-increasing quantity of drugs to produce the higher levels of dopamine required to achieve the "feel good" state. This explains why people "habituate" to drugs, gradually developing a tolerance to the effects of the drugs so that they have to use successively higher doses to achieve the same "high." Any drug addict will tell you that he spends his life chasing that first high.

Cocaine and methamphetamine

Let's turn to the effect cocaine and methamphetamine have on the exposed newborn. As discussed, cocaine produces a "high" by blocking the reuptake of dopamine into the proximal nerve ending, while methamphetamine triggers a high by stimulating excess release of dopamine; the result in both situations is increased availability of dopamine at the distal nerve ending, heightening the excitability of the nerves. This excess dopamine can interfere with blood flow across the placenta from the mother to the fetus, resulting in poor fetal growth, and can cause contractions of the uterus, producing premature labor.

The short-term toxic effects of cocaine and methamphetamine use also bear relation to the high circulating levels of dopamine in the bloodstream. Dopamine acts directly on smooth muscle of the heart and the vascular system, producing a rapid heart rate and constriction of arteries throughout the body with an accompanying acute rise in blood pressure and possible heart attack or stroke. In addition, the excess release of dopamine contributes to dangerous elevations of body temperature and convulsions that can occur during the use of these drugs.

Chronic exposure to cocaine or methamphetamine can result in the "down regulation" of the neurotransmitter receptors. Positron-emission tomography (PET) scans of adults with a long history of use of either of these substances have shown an absence of functioning dopamine receptors in the prefrontal cerebral cortex—the regulatory area of the brain that controls impulsive and aggressive behavior. Animal studies have shown that prenatal exposure to cocaine alters the availability of neurotransmitters in the motor, limbic, and sensory systems, which results in difficulty regulating responses. All this suggests that prenatal exposure to cocaine or methamphetamine has long-term effects on the function of the central nervous system, in general, and on behavioral regulation, specifically.

Newborns who have been prenatally exposed to cocaine or methamphetamine may suffer a range of physical problems, often based on the interruption of adequate blood flow to developing organs in utero. Exposure during gestation can result in babies being born missing a limb or kidney or with a bowel infarction (i.e., death of a portion of the bowel). Cerebral or cardiac infarction—stroke or heart attack—also has been reported in babies whose mothers used cocaine or methamphetamine during pregnancy, especially in instances in which mothers used these drugs during the third trimester. In fact, in some instances heart attacks have been reported *after* birth in infants whose mothers used cocaine just prior to delivery.

Muscle tone in cocaine or methamphetamine-exposed infants can vary; it is not uncommon to see increased tone, resulting in tremulousness and arching behaviors. Such muscle tone problems also may cause feeding difficulties, with poor coordination of the muscles involved in sucking and swallowing. In addition, prenatal exposure to cocaine or methamphetamine may interfere with the infant's neurobehavior—or, the ability of the child to interact with her environment: to respond to sound and visual stimulation, and to engage appropriately with her parents or other caretaker. While physical difficulties occur in only about 25% to 30% of infants exposed prenatally to cocaine or methamphetamine, neurobehavioral difficulties are far more common; it is these latter effects that are the basis of many of the more difficult challenges a parent may confront in caring for the infant.

The cocaine- or methamphetamine-exposed newborn with neuro-behavioral difficulties easily can become overloaded and have difficulty regulating behavior. Sudden changes in light or sound may disrupt his sleep, and he will demonstrate frequent startle reactions and changes in color as he becomes over-stimulated. Communication between parent and child is a two-way street, and the rapidity of the changes in the infant's state of responsiveness significantly disrupts interactions he will have with the parent, adding to the long-term risk.

Environmental methamphetamine exposure

Special mention is required regarding children who live in homes in which methamphetamine is being used or produced. In a

1996–99 report from the Hazardous Substances Emergency Events Surveillance system, 155 persons were found to be injured by exposure to methamphetamine production. Of those injured, 79 were first responders conducting or responding to a methamphetamine laboratory raid: police officers, EMTs, firefighters and hospital employees. Of these, 54% had respiratory irritation, difficulty breathing, and throat irritation. Another 11% had eye irritation. Of the first responders who were injured, the great majority had not worn protective suits at the time of injury. Thus, it is with good reason that fire departments require the use of heavy protective equipment with ventilation systems for first responders when entering a methamphetamine laboratory site.

However, children living in a home with a methamphetamine laboratory do not have the benefit of such protective equipment. They also are exceedingly vulnerable to the hazards of the drug. Children breathe faster than adults, have a faster heartbeat, are smaller and closer to the ground, and have a nervous system that is still developing. In methamphetamine labs, the food children eat is often on the same counter as the site of drug production, and the chemicals used to produce the drug frequently are stored in the refrigerator. Toxicology studies of food taken from home labs have documented significant levels of methamphetamine.

The Centers for Disease Control and Prevention analyzed eight laboratory raids in which thirteen injured children, two to eight years old, were found in the homes. The most common methods of injury to the children were from volatilization due to chemical spills, or fire or explosion due to the unstable combination of the chemicals. A total of four exposures involved anhydrous ammonia; respiratory distress was diagnosed in three of these children. The children had chronic infections and untreated medical conditions. One child had chemical burns from acid exposure. Almost all the children had a positive urine toxicology for methamphetamine.

In a retrospective chart review in Colorado, evaluation was conducted on 76 children younger than age thirteen who were removed from active clandestine methamphetamine laboratories. In this group of children, 9% were found to be anemic, most likely from iron deficiency. Serum chemistries in general were normal except for some level of acidosis found in 27 of the children. Of the 59 children who had a urine toxicology performed, 71% had a positive urine test for methamphetamine or pseudoephedrine/ephedrine, a chemical used in the production of methamphetamine. Ongoing research is evaluating the short and long-term implications of environmental exposure to methamphetamine, but clearly children with such exposure must be observed very carefully as they grow and develop.

Marijuana

Marijuana does not have a direct health effect on pregnancy; there is no increased rate of preterm labor, growth retardation, or other such complications. However, a woman who uses marijuana is more likely to have used other substances including alcohol, tobacco, and other illegal drugs. More importantly, even though marijuana does not affect pregnancy outcome, it does have an impact on fetal brain development. Long-term studies document that children whose mothers have used marijuana during pregnancy have a higher rate of executive functioning difficulties, which interfere with learning and behavior, especially as related to planning and following through with a task.

Tobacco

Tobacco is one of the most harmful substances a woman can use during pregnancy. Among its range of effects, it produces a very high rate of low birth weight, prematurity, and health problems in the newborn and child. The rate of sudden infant death syndrome (SIDS) (crib death) is increased in infants whose mothers smoked tobacco during pregnancy or who are exposed to cigarette smoke in the home after birth. In addition, a woman who admits to using tobacco during pregnancy also is more likely to have used alcohol or illegal drugs. In general, some of the most significant damage from intrauterine tobacco exposure shows up years later; children who were exposed to tobacco in the womb have a significantly higher rate of ADHD as they reach school age and beyond.

In the past two decades, more and more information has emerged about the harm to children's health from environmental tobacco smoke exposure. A 2006 report of the Surgeon General estimated exposure to environmental tobacco smoke at home or in the workplace increases a nonsmoker's risk of developing heart disease by 25% to 30% and lung cancer by 20% to 30%. The U.S. Environmental Protection Agency has classified environmental tobacco smoke a group a human carcinogen, concluding that existing evidence in epidemiologic studies supports a cause-and-effect relationship between exposure and cancer. Among children, for whom the adverse health conditions associated with environmental tobacco smoke exposure are the most severe, environmental exposure has been linked with poor lung growth, exacerbations of asthma, higher rates of lower respiratory illness during the first year of life, acute and recurrent middle ear infections, low birth weight, and SIDS. In fact, a recent large study of approximately 2.5 million live births recorded in Sweden from 1978 to 2004 showed that the risk for SIDS is almost seven times higher than the general population if the mother uses alcohol, tobacco, and/or illicit drugs, and it is more than nine times higher if both parents have a substance use disorder.

Heroin and other opiates

The use of heroin and other opiates has waxed and waned over the last several decades, but opiates once again are emerging as a major substance of abuse. No matter what form the opiate may take—whether it is heroin for intravenous injection, methadone used legally or illegally, or Vicodin or Oxycontin in the form of a prescription drug—abuse can result in the physical dependence of both the mother and the fetus. The newborn infant after birth goes through withdrawal, known as neonatal abstinence syndrome, which mimics narcotic abstinence in an adult. The most significant features of the neonatal abstinence syndrome (Table 3.1) are a high-pitched cry, sweating, tremulousness, scratching of the skin, vomiting, and diarrhea.

TABLE 3.1 NEONATAL ABSTINENCE SYNDROME	
Neurological signs	• Hypertonia • Tremors • Hyperreflexia • Irritability and restlessness • High-pitched cry • Sleep disturbances • Seizures
Autonomic system dysfunction	• Yawning • Nasal stuffiness • Sweating • Sneezing • Low-grade fever • Skin mottling
Gastrointestinal abnormalities	• Diarrhea • Vomiting • Poor feeding • Regurgitation • Swallowing problems • Failure to thrive
Respiratory signs	• Tachypnea • Apnea
Neurobehavioral abnormalities	• Irritability • Poor response to auditory/visual stimulation
Miscellaneous	• Scratching of the skin

Symptoms of neonatal withdrawal from opiates may be present at birth but they usually do not appear until three to four days of life. However, withdrawal depends on many factors, and symptoms may not appear until ten to fourteen days after birth. The withdrawal symptoms peak around six weeks of age and can persist for four to six months or longer. The infants also may demonstrate many of the same problems as other prenatally exposed infants, including low birth weight, prematurity, muscle tone changes, and infant behavioral problems.

When discussing opiate use during pregnancy, it is important to at least briefly mention methadone treatment for narcotic addiction. Methadone is a synthetic narcotic that is used to treat individuals, including pregnant women, who are addicted to heroin, opium, or other narcotics. The advantage of methadone treatment is that it usually requires only one oral dose each day to suppress the desire to use heroin. The risk for infection with the human immunodeficiency virus (HIV) that causes AIDS or with forms of hepatitis is reduced when the pregnant woman is on methadone rather than continuing to use heroin or other narcotics. However, it is important to be aware that infants whose mothers are on methadone during pregnancy can undergo the same difficulties as infants whose mothers continue to use heroin throughout the pregnancy, especially if the mother is on more than 40 milligrams per day in the third trimester.

4　Lake Effect Snow

Marty is a delightful young man, fourteen years old, outgoing, friendly, an excited and excitable child by nature. But Marty has fetal alcohol syndrome, with an IQ in the mid-50s, classic and severe brain changes evidenced on MRI, and rapidly escalating behaviors that drive his adoptive parents to distraction.

Because Marty and his family are in our clinic on a weekly basis for therapy, visiting teams of clinicians frequently meet him. A classic encounter goes this way: Marty enters the conference room and moves directly to the visitors, touching them, looking them in the eye, and saying, "Hi." His greetings won't stop until he has made contact with every person in the room. He then proceeds to inanimate objects—touching, smelling, and in some cases licking various items, all the while smiling and chattering in his private and unfathomable language. Once satisfied, he moves to the front of the room, ready to enjoy the attention from all the new visitors. After a brief conversation with the clinicians, and with some effort on my part, Marty is shepherded out of the room.

"What's his diagnosis?" I ask, as I turn to our visitors. "ADHD!" they respond in chorus. "Did you see the impulsivity, the high level of activity, the distractibility?" These are the same thoughts that Marty's first grade teacher had when she reported that Marty was exhibiting uncontrollable behaviors—coming into the classroom and proceeding to touch every child and every piece of classroom equipment, a whirling dervish in short pants. When the teacher tried to get him to stop and sit down, he resisted. When she moved to restrain him physically, he lashed out and struck her repeatedly. The school demanded he be placed on Ritalin to treat his ADHD before they would allow him back in the classroom.

But is Ritalin the answer? Marty does meet clinical criteria for ADHD, but the source of his behavior eludes the customary treatment. Marty has significant sensory-processing difficulties, expressed through sensory-seeking behaviors. When faced with a new situation, Marty requires as much sensory input as he can gather to find his place in the world. Here the teacher's efforts at restraining him led only to greater frustration on Marty's part, and the only way he knew how to respond was by lashing out. As he fought back, the situation escalated rapidly. Placing Marty on Ritalin to enhance dopamine release in the prefrontal cortex would only have made him more hyper. But if we instead allow Marty to meet his sensory needs through a structured regimen in the classroom, we avoid medication while restricting him as little as possible. In working closely with Marty's special education teacher, this strategy has worked, and now, seven years later, Marty is an endearing child who makes people smile.

Growing up in Texas I had little knowledge of snow other than what I read in the *Bobbsey Twins* book series. Moving to Chicago in the mid-seventies disabused me of any fantasies of the romantic aspects of snowstorms, and by now I have become quite a student of the varieties of snow. The Eskimo language is most descriptive in this regard, with, by some accounts, over one hundred words for snow: *aput* is the root for "snow on the ground," *gana* indicates "falling snow," *piqsirpoq*, "drifting snow," and *qimuqsuq*, "a snow drift."

While the Eskimo language has multiple words for snow's location and form, Chicagoans pride themselves on recognizing the source of snowstorms. Snow driven by the fierce winds of the Northwest falls heavily and horizontally. On the other hand, lake effect snow, caused by climate differences between the land and the relatively warmer waters of Lake Michigan, meanders and drifts on its way to the ground. Though the snow will eventually land, the flakes coming off the lake will first get tossed, turned, pushed and pulled in a variety of directions, creating a pattern of swirling white crystals in the cold air.

Children with sensory integration difficulties share the chaotic, drifting quality of lake effect snow. The structural and functional changes that occur in the developing fetal brain as a result of prenatal substance exposure disrupt sensory pathways. The children know where they need to be but get distracted, preoccupied, and perplexed as they are buffeted by changes in the flow of sensory information from the environment.

Interestingly, in my early work in the 1980s with pregnant women using cocaine, many of the women would tell me that, when high on cocaine, they had a sense of floating; they could not tell where their body ended and the rest of the world began. Newborns prenatally exposed to cocaine often exhibited a similar kind of disorientation. When I undressed the newborn infant and laid him on his back, instead of drawing in his arms and legs to a comforting, midline position, the baby would flail, arms and legs extending frantically, searching for his place in space. This was my earliest recognition of the sensory difficulties young children may have when prenatally exposed to a mother's drugs of abuse.

Sensory integration

Stated simply, sensory integration refers to the process through which the brain understands, organizes, interprets, and integrates the sensory information we receive from the world around us so that we can make use of the information in our lives. Sensations such as movement, body awareness, touch, sight, sound, and the pull of gravity make up the overall sensory experience. Information from the environment is received by our senses and sent to the corresponding regions of the brain where it is interpreted and organized. All of the senses work together to form an overall conceptualization of what is happening to us and around us.

Sensory integration comprises four steps:

1. *Input* — bringing information into the brain along the appropriate pathway. Each type of information travels along a different nerve pathway to be recorded in a distinct part of the brain. Visual information travels from the eye along the optic nerve to insert in the occipital lobe at the back of the brain. Touch and taste enter through the parietal lobe; smell goes directly to the thalamus. Sound enters through the ear and is transported along the auditory nerve to insert in the midline of the brain.

2. *Integration* — consolidating the information. A primary job of the brain is to integrate the sensory information to create a smooth interplay of all the senses.

3. *Memory* — storing the information for later use. Information is stored as memory and perceptions until the time—either immediate or delayed—when the information is needed. When necessary, the information is conducted forward to the prefrontal cortex, where dopamine and other key neurotransmitters are stored.

4. *Output* — using the information to guide the use of language and motor skills so an individual is able to respond appropriately. The prefrontal cortex is the regulatory center of the brain, where neurotransmitters such as dopamine, serotonin, and norepinephrine fire off to regulate actions, behavior, emotion, and speech and language.

Sensory input arrives via the five basic senses that feed us information from the environment: tactile (touch), gustatory (taste), visual (sight), auditory (sound), and olfactory (smell). But there are two other less-known sources of sensory information: proprioception and vestibular. Proprioception uses unconscious input from muscles and joints to allow us to know where our body is in relation to other body parts and in relation to other objects in the environment. It also signals to us how our body is moving. Because of its function in estimating the movement of our bodies, proprioception plays a critical role in keeping us from physical harm, such as bumping into the table as we walk through a room. In addition, it helps us avoid social gaffes by allowing us to judge and keep appropriate physical distance from others while engaged in conversation.

Vestibular input is important for control of balance. Received from receptors in the inner ear, vestibular input lets us know where the head is in relation to the body, how gravity is affecting us, and whether we are moving or standing still. It also lets us know in what direction we are moving, and just how fast we are going.

It is easy to take sensory integration for granted since it occurs naturally, as sensory needs are met through everyday activities and socially acceptable behaviors.

TABLE 4.1 COMMON SIGNS OF SENSORY-PROCESSING DYSFUNCTION

- Clumsy
- Over- or under-sensitive to sounds, sights, smell, touch, or movement
- Distractible
- Unusually active at either a high or low level of activity
- Hard to calm down
- Difficulty during transitions and struggles to adapt to changes in routine
- Picky when eating — particularly sensitive to the texture or feel of foods
- Resistant to touching things — e.g., resists going barefoot in the grass, playing in the sand
- Defensive to light touch
- Very agitated when spinning or roughhousing
- Likely to seek out excessive spinning or swinging
- Prone to exhibit rocking or swaying body movements
- Overly excited during play to the point that he cannot calm down
- Aware of noises that others do not notice
- Unusually difficult during teeth brushing, hair washing, and bathing
- Sensitive to clothing textures and tags
- Unable to fall or stay asleep

Children use play—running, climbing, jumping, swinging—to fulfill their sensory needs. They crunch on carrot sticks, sit in rocking chairs, and crawl across grass. Together these everyday activities constitute a normal sensory experience, and contribute to a child's motor planning abilities and ability to adapt to changing situations. Successful sensory experiences during childhood provide a crucial foundation for later, more complex learning and behavior. Proper sensory integration helps a child maintain attention and build positive relationships with others. Ultimately, sensory integration contributes to the healthy development of the child's self-esteem and ability to learn and concentrate.

However exposure to alcohol or illicit drugs during the prenatal period can disrupt sensory processing. As we have seen earlier, the limbic system, which serves a central organizing and transmitting function in sensory integration, lies in the exact midline of the brain, making it a primary target for alcohol toxicity. The child who has been exposed to alcohol in early gestation is set up for deficits in sensory-processing capabilities; he is like that snowflake off Lake Michigan, pushed and pulled in multiple directions at once.

Sensory-processing dysfunction

Sensory processing allows us to use information from the environment to guide motor, emotional, and language functioning in appropriate response to the environment. However, damage to the limbic system due to alcohol exposure or damage to the prefrontal cortex by illicit drugs or tobacco interferes with the way the child interprets and uses the information. This disruption limits the child's ability to process sensory cues from his environment. One should bear in mind that the existence of a *sensory-processing deficit* does not necessarily imply prenatal substance exposure: several other factors may contribute to the development of sensory-processing problems. Children who experience premature birth, environmental neglect, brain injury, autism, or other developmental disorders are more likely to have difficulty managing sensory information. In many instances, there is no identifiable cause for the child's sensory-processing problems.

Dysfunction may show up in several ways. If a child cannot filter information as it comes in to the brain, the brain quickly becomes overloaded and causes the child to avoid sensory stimuli. Conversely, when there is a problem integrating and organizing sensory information, the brain receives too little input and seeks out additional sensory information. If a child cannot "read" his body in order to know where he is in relation to other objects, he is off balance and poorly coordinated; he is labeled as "accident prone" or, simply, a klutz.

At times the problems of sensory integration and processing deficits can become very complicated. Some children with prenatal substance exposure may have higher sensory thresholds, and others may have lower sensory thresholds. When the child has a higher threshold, as is true for Marty, our case study at the outset of the chapter, he may be under-sensitive to sensory stimulation; he requires greater amounts of sensory stimulation for the input to register. For example, when a child has a higher threshold for auditory stimuli, he may not register someone speaking in a normal speaking voice. Rather, the speaker may need to raise his voice before the child is actually able to perceive it. This may be frustrating for adults who feel they are being ignored and constantly having to yell at their child; however, the real difficulty for the child is not inattention but inability to process auditory information.

Children with lower sensory thresholds may exhibit distractible and irritable behaviors that interfere with academics, play, and social relationships. For example, a child with a lower threshold for auditory stimuli would be overly sensitive to sounds. Because of this sensitivity, the child may be bothered by noises so quiet they do not even register for other children. The child not only may take note of background noises others filter out, but may drift off task due to noises that occupy her attention, disrupting her ability to perform academically.

A child with a sensory-processing deficit — whether the child is under- or oversensitive — often appears disorganized. She has difficulty incorporating into the brain all of the input received from the environment and making sense out of it. The child may look distracted or fidgety and have difficulty responding appropriately to the input she receives. As a coping mechanism, a child with a sensory-processing deficit will attempt to normalize her nervous system. If the child is oversensitive and input is constantly overwhelming to her she will be sensory-avoidant. She will cover her ears at noises that are tolerable to others, spit out food with a texture she cannot tolerate, or cling to her parent in a crowded store. On the other hand, some children may make up for a sensory-processing deficit by being sensory-seeking: they seek out input to normalize their nervous system. They may bang toys to create noise, touch everything in sight, or flick light switches to create a more intense visual spectacle. It is easy to see how a sensory-seeking child could easily be labeled as "hyperactive."

Children who are experiencing sensory integration difficulties are not intentionally misbehaving. They simply are trying to gain the additional input that their body needs or, conversely, attempting to avoid extra stimulation in order to function properly. Often these children are intelligent and capable, but struggle to control their body and their need to manage sensory inputs. It is important to remember that the sensory needs of these children are just that — needs. Trying to diminish the needs for these behaviors will not be effective, but finding adaptable ways to satisfy the sensory needs of the child can be effective. Giving the child a way to acquire necessary sensory stimulation, such as with a simple "fidget toy," eliminates his need to find sensory input through more disruptive behavior. Eliminating sensory overload allows the child to remain calm and on task, less conscious of distracters from the environment.

It must be noted that many of the behaviors discussed in this section occur normally, especially in preschool and elementary school children. The range of normal behavior is wide and varied:

pushing, biting, fear, and social anxiety can all be part of the profile of a normally developing child. However, persistent patterns of behavior, such as chronically seeking out heightened sensation — slamming doors, flicking lights, hitting or biting oneself, screaming for no purpose — may indicate that the child is experiencing poor sensory processing. Frequency, intensity, and duration are critical to distinguish normal from worrisome behavior. Children with sensory integration problems exhibit these behaviors multiple times a day, in an extreme manner, for several minutes or longer. These behaviors cannot be viewed in isolation, but need to be looked at as part of a pattern.

Sensory integration therapy

Just as a parent would not punish a child for being unable to run swiftly, the child experiencing sensory difficulties should not be punished for behavioral traits beyond his control. Most often the child's behavior is merely an attempt to normalize his nervous system. Sensory integration therapy attempts to bring sensory input into alignment for the child. If a child is suspected of having difficulty with one or more of his sensory systems, an evaluation by an occupational therapist trained in sensory integration issues is necessary to determine if the child is experiencing sensory-processing difficulties. Although most occupational therapists are aware of sensory integration and the effects it has on behavior, special training is required before an occupational therapist is qualified to provide sensory integration treatment. Speech-language pathologists also may have training in this area, although they concentrate on the child's oral motor sensitivities and how these affect the child's feeding and speaking.

Sensory integration therapy is child centered and focuses on the child's specific needs. As the child's skill level increases, the therapy curriculum is modified to accommodate the progress. Like any therapy regimen, sensory integration therapy is most beneficial if the recommended strategies are incorporated into a child's daily environment. No treatment is effective if practiced for only an hour or a half-hour each week. Parents of children in sensory integration therapy should attend the treatment sessions with the child's therapist and follow through with exercises throughout the week. Learning to recognize cues of sensory needs is important to help the child learn to regulate his own system, and a good therapist will offer practical strategies that parents can practice with their child in order to maximize the effectiveness of the treatment. For example, early in therapy a child will need to be told when it is time to go to his quiet chair in order to have some "cool down" time. The time spent in the quiet area should not be punitive for the child, but should signal to the child that his behavior is inappropriate. Eventually, the child will learn to recognize cues that he is becoming overwhelmed, and he will go to the cool down area without the direction of his parent or teacher.

Sensory integration strategies for the home

Every child who is having trouble with sensory integration is different, but there are general strategies families can use to help the child. A common metaphor used by sensory integration therapists is the sensory diet: in other words, the list of strategies chosen to "feed" the sensory needs of a child with sensory integration dysfunction. While a sensory diet may include a list of foods that can help a child to regulate behavior, foods are certainly not the only items on the sensory "diet" list. The sensory diet includes all activities and environmental modifications that can be tailored to the specific needs of a child's sensory system. Remember, the strategies in Table 4.2 will need to be reinforced until a child learns to use the strategies himself to regulate behavior.

While Table 4.2 includes some of the more common strategies families use to provide their children with necessary sensory input, there is also a wide range of strategies not listed that may be right for a particular child. Some children will love certain approaches and not be able to tolerate others. It is vital to find what works (and what doesn't) for the child's sensory needs. In advising parents, I recommend they work closely with a therapist trained in sensory integration to customize a sensory diet that will work for the child.

The Wilbarger Deep Pressure and Propioceptive Technique (DPPT) & Oral Tactile Technique (OTT) developed by Patricia Wilbarger, an occupational therapist and clinical psychologist, is another available treatment method that has demonstrated success. To perform this technique the trained therapist or parent applies firm strokes on the child's limbs and back with a soft, non-scratching pressure brush. The brushing is combined with deep pressure to the joints. Many parents report that their child seems more organized after the brushing/joint compressions. The DPPT & OTT technique must be performed with the guidance of an occupational therapist in order to learn the proper technique and to monitor the child's response.

Once a parent figures out techniques that work for a child, the next step is to make sure the techniques are actually available. Many older children carry a "sensory backpack" filled with tools to regulate their system. For younger children, it is crucial for teachers or caregivers to get involved and have sensory diet items handy for the child to use throughout the day.

Every child is different. If you attempt a treatment strategy that does not work to fulfill the child's sensory needs, it is okay to try something else. Be patient with the child and keep in mind that the difficult behaviors are not willful. The child is not acting out of spite. She is exhibiting the behaviors because of a neurologically based drive to regulate her nervous system. The best support a parent or therapist can offer is informed and patient guidance in helping the child find the sensory diet that will work for her.

To appreciate what a child with sensory integration dysfunction goes through on a daily basis, just think of sitting in on one of the recent 3-D movies that are all the rage. The purpose of these movies is to enhance sensory input. Now imagine if in that same movie the sound were turned up twice as high and three times as many objects

TABLE 4.2 MODIFICATIONS FOR A CHILD WITH A SENSORY-PROCESSING DEFICIT	
• Provide deep pressure input (as taught by an occupational therapist) to joints and large muscles	• Use firm touch for organization, such as a bear hug or hand placement on the child's shoulders
• Give a massage with or without lotion	• Provide a body pillow for sleeping
• Provide a miniature trampoline for jumping	• Tuck in sheets or blankets tightly
• Have the child pull a heavy wagon or push a heavy buggy	• Encourage swinging, rocking, or gliding, when appropriate
• Cover the child in bed with a heavy or weighted blanket or place it in his lap while sitting	• Encourage the child to discreetly perform many small stretching exercises at his school desk
• Provide acceptable fidget toys, such as bracelets, textured stickers on books, key chains, squishy pencil grips, or squeezable objects for use inside pockets	• Let the child do heavy work: lifting, carrying groceries, scrubbing floors, transferring laundry from washer to dryer, pushing the vacuum
• Create a "cool down" area free of excessive distractions	• Use sun visors if the child is very disturbed by bright lights
• Use a white noise machine or fan at night	• Try different textures for sheets and pillowcases
• Use ear plugs if the child is very disturbed or distracted by loud sounds	• Find the appropriate "hug level" that works for both the child and the parent

were flying toward your cardboard 3-D eyewear. This is the feeling of constant assault under which many alcohol- and drug-exposed children find themselves. Just as the snowflake on Lake Michigan is tossed and turned by swirling winds, just as Marty can't find enough information to guide behavior and thought, children with sensory integration deficits can get lost in their journey toward the desired goal.

TABLE 4.2 (*continued*) MODIFICATIONS FOR A CHILD WITH A SENSORY-PROCESSING DEFICIT	
• Introduce textures gradually — children may be willing to first explore a texture such as shaving cream, beans or sand inside a plastic bag before gradually allowing the substance to touch their skin	• Be aware of intrusive clothing seams or itchy tags — after a while we don't even notice they are there, but a child with sensory integration issues will be bothered the entire day
• Use loose clothing one size too large or with an elastic waist; or use tight tee shirts, such as a spandex blend, under clothing	• Use a firm pillow or tightly rolled towel, at the top of the bed, to push against for gentle head pressure
• Encourage oral activities that are calming: chewing gum, using a water bottle with a straw, chewing on a straw, blowing a cotton ball through a straw, eating sour candy and chewy or crunchy foods	• Experiment with scents such as vanilla, almond, coconut, grape, lavender or citrus; if these are calming, they can be applied to clothing or pillowcases
• Create a "cool down" area free of excessive distractions	• Find the appropriate "hug level" that works for both the child and the parent
• Set up an obstacle course that allows for jumping, climbing, and tunneling during play time	• Allow a child who needs frequent breaks to deliver notes to the school office or to retrieve supplies

Special note: *Do not take away playtime or recess privileges as a punishment for disruptive behavior. Activities during recess such as running, jumping, swinging and sliding are essential to help regulate the child's sensory system. Depriving a child of the input he receives during recess or similar gross motor activities may increase problematic behaviors.*

5 Through the Looking Glass

I think I should understand that better, if I had it written down: but I can't quite follow it as you say it.
— Lewis Carroll, *Alice's Adventures in Wonderland*

Carlos is charged with murder. At fourteen years of age, he was found, gun in hand, on a hill overlooking a country road running through an Indian reservation. A driver had just been shot through the head. When the police questioned him immediately afterward, he readily confessed to having pulled the trigger.

Two years later he is still in juvenile lock-up, charged as an adult. A new defense attorney, recently assigned the case, has begun to find inconsistencies in the story. In meeting with Carlos's grandparents and extended family, she learned that his mother has been shunned by the rest of the Native American community because of her relentless drinking and methamphetamine use, uninterrupted throughout her many pregnancies. Carlos has bounced from one relative's home to another, but the child welfare system has never found cause to officially remove him from his birth home.

School reports portray Carlos as socially isolated and sad. Academically, he has failed in almost every subject. Teachers describe him as disorganized, easily confused, and susceptible to the harsh put-downs aimed his way by other students. Previous evaluations of Carlos have revealed an IQ of 72 and led to diagnoses ranging from

ADHD to conduct disorder, to posttraumatic stress disorder.

I met Carlos in an eight-by-eight-foot locked room painted a drab green and smudged by years of pounding, tear-stained hands. The linoleum floor was cracked and warped, and the round table that separated us wobbled on the uneven ground. The single source of light was a high window, allowing a small square of sunlight into the room.

Carlos met my gaze momentarily, but then averted his eyes as if any human connection were too much for him to tolerate. His round face showed no signs of prenatal alcohol exposure, and his shy smile communicated only feelings of loss.

Neurologically, Carlos was intact. He showed only mild deficits in fine motor skills. As we talked, he began to open up, and it wasn't long before he was speaking of his experiences at juvenile hall. Throughout the conversation, it was clear his thoughts didn't always connect, and his ability to express complex ideas was severely limited. On simple tests of sequencing, he could complete no more than one-step commands at a time. Anything that required holding a series of thoughts in his head was lost in confusion. During these moments his frustration showed with increasing agitation, but he would then quickly collect himself and put up a show of bravado.

Carlos has yet to go to trial, and it remains to be seen what will happen to him. The facts against him are damning: his fingerprints were on the murder weapon and he confessed to the crime. Still, through our conversation a story emerged that, if true, jeopardizes the evidence of Carlos's having pulled the trigger. Carlos was present at the time of the shooting, a case of a drug deal gone bad. The shooter turned to Carlos after firing the fatal shot and handed the gun to Carlos. "Hold this for me, will ya'," he said. Carlos, eager to please, took the gun. As he told me

in the interview, "I thought the cops wanted me to say
yes when they asked me if I shot the guy, so I said, yes."

Although Carlos's story is extreme, within it we find the worry of
every adoptive parent: "What does the future hold?" The simple
answer . . . we don't know.

Under normal circumstances, children undergo an exciting
period of development from the ages four through six. As their
cognitive abilities develop, they are able to speak in complete
sentences and begin to articulate what they are learning: they begin
to count, label pictures and colors, and recognize shapes. Physically,
they are able to walk on their toes, climb ladders, and use their
notion of balance to ride a bike. They learn skills such as running,
kicking, and throwing a ball which allow them to interact socially
with peers. Due to increased fine motor control, they are able to
hold a pencil well enough to draw shapes; they learn to write, dress
themselves, and complete simple chores around the house. While
younger toddlers typically show a casual interest in peers and play
alongside one another without interacting, four- to six-year-olds
begin to revel in playing and interacting with their peers; they start
to engage in more cooperative play and show increased interest in
imaginary activity, whether it is playing house or slaying dragons.

As children get older, they experience changes in their
body, mind, and sense of self-identity that require significant
psychological adjustment. Normal adolescence is characterized
by a lengthy transition period in which the adolescent is neither
a child nor an adult. Although most adolescents cope successfully
with the developmental demands of this period, adolescence does
tend to generate more turmoil than any other stage of development.
The transition from childhood to adulthood is characterized by
dramatic changes in identity, self-consciousness, and cognitive
flexibility, and is not easy under the best of circumstances.

The notion that the brain continues to develop after childhood
is relatively new. One particular region, the prefrontal cortex,

undergoes significant changes during puberty and adolescence. This brain region is responsible for executive functioning; specifically, how we orchestrate thoughts and actions in accordance with internal goals. Executive functioning is involved in planning complex cognitive behaviors and expressing one's personality. It allows individuals to differentiate among conflicting thoughts and filter out unimportant information. It also helps us anticipate future consequences of current activities, work toward a defined goal, and inhibit impulses that could lead to socially unacceptable outcomes.

Many MRI studies have demonstrated developmental changes in the prefrontal cortex during adolescence that support the theory that adolescence is a time of improvement in executive functioning skills. For example, selective attention, decision making, and inhibition skills, along with the ability to carry out multiple tasks at once, each usually improve during adolescence. On the other hand, adolescents with alcohol and drug exposure have been shown to demonstrate difficulties with information processing and memory tasks, as well as self-regulation and planning, all important components of executive functioning.

Because childhood — all the way through adolescence — is a time of such rapid and amazing transformation, it is difficult to look at a child at any one point in time and predict what lies down the road. However, the following discussion attempts a generalized look at what we know about the impact of prenatal alcohol and illicit drug exposure on the long-term outcome of the child. Throughout the discussion, be aware that there are very few children in this world that are exposed to only cocaine or *only* methamphetamine or *only* alcohol during pregnancy. As previously discussed, women tend to be polydrug users, which means that the fetus is exposed to a host of substances during critical phases of brain development. Barring an unforeseen breakthrough in research methods, we will never be able to securely attach any one specific finding to one specific substance. With that in mind, we will use the term "substance-exposed" for those difficulties associated with a broad range of substances; in cases when the research findings are isolated to a single substance, we will name that substance specifically. Accepting the limitations of the evidence at hand, let us examine the impact of prenatal alcohol and drug exposure on long-term child development, learning, and behavior.

Cognitive development

The first thing to remember about cognitive development in substance-exposed children is there is quite a bit of difference between children exposed prenatally to alcohol and those exposed to illicit drugs. In alcohol-exposed children, there are reports of lower developmental scores from as early as eight months of age. While these findings did not hold up at 18 months of age, the same children were retested at 51 months of age, utilizing the Wechsler Preschool and Primary Test of Intelligence, and at that point lower IQ scores were indeed related to higher levels of prenatal alcohol exposure.

Young infants exposed to alcohol during the gestational period are particularly vulnerable to damage to areas of the brain responsible for intellectual functioning. These infants may be slow to process and respond to various kinds of stimulation and may perform poorly in directed activities and sustained play. The brain's slower and less efficient information processing also has implications for the older child and may show up as an apparent difficulty in concept development, abstract functioning, or higher-level executive functioning, or give rise to learning disabilities.

As the alcohol-exposed children grow older, cognitive deficits can become more obvious. In one study, four-year-old children who had been exposed to alcohol were three times more likely to have an IQ score below 85 if they had been exposed to 3 or more drinks per day in utero. This study also noted that the children had the most difficulty in tasks requiring perceptual organization, attention to visual detail, working memory, math skills, and executive functioning.

At school age, IQ scores in alcohol-exposed children tend to fall in the mildly impaired to borderline range. However, many children with prenatal exposure to alcohol have satisfactory cognitive abilities. One study comparing the neuropsychological results of early school-age children with varied durations of prenatal alcohol exposure found that the average IQ scores of all subgroups (children exposed to alcohol in the first trimester, children exposed to alcohol in the first and second trimesters, and children exposed to alcohol throughout the pregnancy) were within the average range. The only exception was found in verbal IQ score, which was measured at just below average for children exposed throughout pregnancy.

Clinical work with alcohol-exposed children confirms that at school age the children may demonstrate a wide range of cognitive abilities. On one extreme, there are those who exhibit significant global delays. On the other end are alcohol-exposed children who display average or even better than average cognitive skills. Still other alcohol-exposed children demonstrate relatively solid cognitive skills with pockets of deficit limited to a specific area or two. But even alcohol-exposed children with average or better cognitive abilities often struggle to apply these abilities in daily living. As they grow into adolescence and older, these children frequently demonstrate difficulty with abstract reasoning and rely, instead, on more concrete thought processes; they often think in terms of "black and white."

> The call came at five in the morning. Mitch had been arrested, charged with breaking and entering. He had given the police my name and cell phone number. It wasn't a necessarily unexpected call. I had known Mitch since his adoption at two weeks of age. Prenatally exposed to alcohol and cocaine, his IQ was in the mid-90s, which gave him an ability to respond well to treatment interventions. He had good global cognitive skills and had made it through high school with the help of a tutor and a committed family that closely monitored his

schoolwork and social life. But following high school, Mitch couldn't hold a job. This was a clear setback, but Mitch persevered. He ended up working for his father, and things were going so well that at the age of nineteen he was about to try living on his own.

Then came Christmas season. Mitch was out with friends when an old acquaintance, a sixteen-year-old girl, invited him to come over to her house sometime "to hang out." That night, at three in the morning, Mitch went to her house. The back door was open, so he proceeded up the stairs, found her bedroom, and shook her out of her sleep. She awoke to the sight of a tall figure looming over her in the dark and began to scream. Her parents came running, threw on the light, and there was Mitch. They called the police; the police called me. "Hey, doc," came the booming voice over the phone. "We got a kid down here, and we're booking him for breaking and entering. And we're really ticked off, 'cause we keep asking him, 'What the hell were you doing banging into that house?' and all he says is 'She invited me over.'"

I went to the police station, preparing Mitch's defense during the car ride. Thankfully, it turned out to be unnecessary. We convinced the family to drop the charges, and Mitch was able to go home with his parents. But to this day, when I talk about this incident with Mitch, who is now twenty-four years old, he looks at me with a hint of puzzlement and says simply, "But she invited me over."

Mitch demonstrates the difficulty many young adults prenatally exposed to alcohol have in applying their knowledge to day-to-day situations and understanding the future outcomes or consequences of their actions. Even in the best of circumstances, typically developing adolescents are poor at decision making, especially when risk is involved. Changes in brain structure and functioning induced by prenatal alcohol exposure further compromise an adolescent's ability to make decisions and often lead to risky, delinquent behavior.

Children exposed prenatally to illicit drugs present a different picture of global cognitive development from children with prenatal alcohol exposure. Though there is no information regarding the long-term impact of methamphetamine use in pregnancy, studies consistently report that prenatal exposure to cocaine, opiates, and other illicit drugs has minimal direct influence on global cognitive development. Further, it is becoming increasingly clear that the key predictor of cognitive development, other than genetics, is the environment in which the child is raised. One study of children prenatally exposed to cocaine and other drugs found that by six years of age, 60% of the children's birth mothers were continuing to use drugs and alcohol. Confoundingly, the most important factor predicting the child's IQ at six years of age was not the child's prenatal exposure but the mother's patterns of drug use after the baby was born. A home in which drugs were used was a home in which the child's needs for intellectual stimulation and developmental support were not met. Drug-exposed foster and adopted children who do not suffer neurological damage in the perinatal period, who have lived in a stable environment, and who have been given the kinds of interventions they required through early childhood exhibit normal global cognitive development. This reiterates the principal of infant mental health: all aspects of a child's development occur within the context of a positive, secure, parent-child relationship.

Memory

Alcohol-exposed children display poorer immediate recall of visual and verbal information than their non-exposed peers. However, in some studies, while children with prenatal alcohol exposure recalled significantly less information than the comparison group of non-exposed children after a brief delay, the alcohol-exposed children retained the same proportion of information as the non-exposed children over the long term. So, while alcohol-exposed children exhibited poorer verbal and visual learning, their relative retention of the material was the same as the matched controls.

Those who work with alcohol-exposed children know that, in addition to general concerns about memory and learning, one of the most common problems reported by parents involves the children's inconsistent memory. Often caregivers express frustration about their child's ability to remember things on some days but not others. Understandably, inconsistencies in recall can be extremely frustrating for parents and teachers. It is important that parents and educators understand that inconsistent storage and recall has origins in the brain-based changes associated with prenatal alcohol exposure and is not a sign of "laziness" or a problem with motivation.

These problems with memory can produce deficits in sustained attention: the ability to remain alert and focused over time. This becomes especially evident on tasks that also require active processing of information. For this reason, staying focused on a reading comprehension test often proves difficult for alcohol-exposed children. Other studies have found deficits in sustained attention tasks that require active recall of information or response inhibition. This evidence suggests that the deficit lies in impairment in executive function rather than sustained attention.

Speech and language

Prenatal substance exposure can impact the young child's speech and language development. In the neonatal period, decreased or increased facial tone and oral motor difficulties contribute not only to feeding problems, but also to long-term deficits in speech and language development. In addition, children who have a high-arched palate, a characteristic of alcohol exposure, often show articulation difficulties as they grow older. Many substance-exposed children, particularly if someone in the home is smoking cigarettes, are susceptible to recurrent ear infections, which can result in delayed language development and phonological problems. Furthermore, alcohol may directly damage the eighth cranial nerve, the auditory nerve, so that many of these children experience auditory sensory sensitivities and in some cases neurosensory hearing loss. Many of these early difficulties with hearing can contribute to decreased attention, and, in turn, to a greater number of acting out behaviors; for when children have difficulty communicating effectively with others, they can experience frustration with themselves and ostracism by peers, resorting to misconduct or delinquency as a result.

Motor development

Prenatal substance exposure can produce problems in integrating and coordinating motor control as well as difficulties with the child's muscle tone (hypotonia or hypertonia or a combination of both). This may lead to delays in both fine and gross motor development and affect early eye-hand coordination in the infant. Ongoing immaturities in the central nervous system appear in delays in the child's development of strength, stability, coordination, and balance. With therapy, many of the children will attain their motor developmental milestones, but they often continue to be clumsy. This can cause problems with the child's ability to plan his motor activities, which can interfere with learning. As the children become increasingly involved in activities that require both gross and fine motor activities, motor skill deficits can have a significant impact on their lives. Participation in sports activities can be especially difficult for children who struggle with gross motor functioning, necessary for running and kicking. Ultimately, problems with motor development may contribute to difficulties with peer relationships, particularly when athletics and sports are highly valued in the child's peer group.

Academic performance

Educationally, children and adolescents who have been exposed to alcohol often display hyperactivity, trouble completing tasks, and a lack of appropriate initiative, all of which impede learning. These children repeatedly fail to complete assignments or schoolwork and have difficulty organizing their materials. Children and adolescents exposed to alcohol or drugs often are labeled "problem children," and are singled out in school due to their disruptive behaviors in the classroom. As prenatal exposure can be a "hidden disability" due to the often subtle physical characteristics it manifests, many of these children are never diagnosed properly and slip through the cracks in the education system.

Math is a particularly difficult subject for children with prenatal substance exposure. One study of older children and adults found that individuals prenatally exposed to alcohol demonstrated poor number processing skills. While the alcohol-exposed children performed as well as non-exposed children on simple math tasks, they had difficulty on more complex tasks that required abstract reasoning. As long as a task was concrete, the children did fine; however, as the math tasks became increasingly complex and abstract, they struggled. Difficulties in working through abstract concepts generalize to other academic areas: the more complex and abstract the work, the more difficult it is for the child to succeed. Consequently, by third grade, when schoolwork increasingly moves from the concrete to the abstract, the child begins to fall further and further behind.

Social skills

Children with prenatal alcohol exposure often struggle socially, with discrepancies between age and age-equivalent social expectations growing each year. Their peers turn away from them as they get older, viewing children exposed to alcohol as immature and "babyish" in their interests. It is important to note that the children are no less socially inclined than their non-exposed peers; they crave friendships and social interactions. One twelve-year-old boy, Micah, with whom I have worked for many years, continuously goes out of his way to strengthen relationships with his fellow seventh-graders, especially the girls. In one instance, he took his mother's diamond earrings out of her jewelry box and gave them to a girl at school. When the girl's mother discovered the gift, she promptly returned them. Micah feels no remorse for the theft, only sadness that the girl still doesn't like him.

Interestingly, the children's cognitive deficits do not play much of a role in their social difficulties; rather it is problems with sensory processing and behavioral regulation that contribute most to social isolation. Children exposed prenatally to alcohol or illicit drugs have sensory deficits that impede their understanding of the concept of personal space. The children constantly cross socially acceptable physical boundaries and are labeled as "aggressive."

Even simple conversations and group interactions are difficult for prenatally exposed children. The majority of the meaning derived from communication comes from nonverbal cues such as facial expression, eye contact, posture, gestures, tone of voice, and physical space: over 90% of communication is nonverbal. Nonverbal cues are subtle, complicated, and abstract. They appear vague and confusing for prenatally exposed children. If the child cannot read nonverbal cues, he may misinterpret or miss out on the majority of information being communicated.

> Angela once again was suspended from school, this time for hitting her classmate, Sheila. What had been a friendly encounter escalated into an unprovoked slugfest when Sheila told Angela she was "bad." In the language of the street, "bad" means hip and savvy; from Sheila's perspective this was meant as high praise. But to understand "bad" as a compliment, Angela had to be able to interpret Sheila's tone of voice, facial expression, and body.

As substance-exposed children approach the developmental transition to adolescence, social relationships become increasingly complex. For the adolescent who already has difficulties interpreting both verbal and nonverbal communication, relationships with peers, caregivers, employers, and romantic partners often prove to be confusing—at times overwhelming. While the relational demands of adolescence increase in complexity, the teen with prenatal alcohol or drug exposure often continues to struggle with difficulties making and keeping friends, perceiving and resisting peer pressure, and feeling accepted within a peer group. This inability to engage in mutually rewarding relationships with one's peers can restrict the adolescent's development of self-identity and impede the young person's future success with relationships.

Over time adolescence is accompanied by maturation of brain functions, increasing a young adult's capacity to think and reason abstractly. However, for adolescents who have problems with abstract thinking as a result of exposure, social problem-solving skills and difficulties with generalization (i.e., the ability to apply what one knows to different situations and to learn from one's mistakes) persist. While teens in general are susceptible to peer influence, the teen with alcohol and drug exposure often lacks the ability to reason effectively in unclear or confusing social situations. Carlos's decision to handle the assailant's murder weapon and Mitchell's decision to enter a girl's home unannounced at three o'clock in the morning are perfect examples. In both cases, the substance exposure interferes with the teen's ability to think things through. That places him at increased risk of being taken advantage of, particularly by individuals who encourage his participation in maladaptive or anti-social behaviors.

Drug- and alcohol-exposed adolescents often have difficulty with self-reflection and do not recognize the impact their behavior has on others and on their environment. If the adolescent cannot reflect on the effect his actions have on those around him, the ability to empathize is inevitably impaired, and he will behave in ways that others perceive as insulting. Worse, he will have a hard time reading the nonverbal cues friends and family members may send to express that they have been hurt or offended. Unfortunately, these difficulties interpreting social cues often are misinterpreted as a lack of empathy or remorse when more often they are a result of social skills deficits related to the exposure.

Adaptive functioning

Adaptive behavior refers to how effectively an individual conforms to life demands: communication, socialization, and daily living skills like brushing teeth. For most children, there is a direct relationship between intellectual functioning and adaptive behavior. However, individuals affected by prenatal exposure to alcohol represent one of the few disability groups in which a significant discrepancy exists between intellectual functioning and adaptive behavior.

As the exposed child transitions into adolescence, she may begin to lag even further behind her peers in the areas of communication, daily living skills, and socialization than she did as a younger child. The combined effects of executive, cognitive, and adaptive functioning deficits interfere with the teen's ability to perform age-expected daily living tasks such as budgeting finances, managing time, taking care of one's personal and hygiene needs, keeping a job, completing daily routines and chores, and following community rules and expectations. Unfortunately, many adolescents with these difficulties simply are labeled as "bad" in communities that do not understand the subtle difficulties that occur within this population. It often is necessary for adults in the adolescent's life to function as the child's "external brain," providing high levels of support, guidance, and supervision, well into adulthood. The ultimate goal for the adolescent remains the internalization of habits and routines that will promote the development of independent living skills. Strong and continued support from the parent or caregiver is a necessary component of proper care for alcohol-exposed teens, and most likely, for those with illicit drug exposure as well.

TABLE 5.1 BEHAVIORAL PATTERNS IN CHILDREN PRENATALLY EXPOSED TO ILLICIT DRUGS	
Anxiety or depression	• Feels the need to be perfect • Feels unloved • Threatened by others • Feels worthless or inferior • Worries excessively
Social problems	• Acts younger than his age • Clings to others • Gets teased frequently • Disliked by other children
Thought problems	• Has recurring thoughts • Repeats particular acts • Stares • Has strange ideas
Attention problems	• Cannot concentrate for long • Cannot sit still • Daydreams often • Acts impulsively • Has difficulty staying on task
Delinquent behavior	• Exhibits little or no guilt after misbehaving • Lies, cheats, or steals
Aggressive behavior	• Argues frequently • Demands attention • Destroys property • Is disobedient and stubborn • Has sudden mood changes • Talks too much and is unusually loud • Has temper tantrums
Poor executive functioning	• Gets lost in conversations • Cannot follow sequenced instructions • Struggles to make decisions

Behavior

By far the most common, and often the most devastating, aspect of long term outcome is the impact prenatal exposure to alcohol and illicit drugs can have on the child's behavior. While, in general, illicit drug exposure does not have a direct effect on the child's intellectual performance, studies do show that children exposed to cocaine, heroin, marijuana, and other drugs, including alcohol, are more likely to have behavioral, emotional, and learning problems in preschool and elementary school. As we will discuss further in chapter 6, a typical behavioral pattern that emerges is ADHD. What is important to understand is that the behaviors these children demonstrate are not necessarily due to willful disobedience, but based in part on damage to the child's neurological system. Table 5.1 provides an overview of the most common problems seen in children who have been prenatally exposed to alcohol or illicit drugs. Remember, no one substance of abuse can be associated with any one particular problem, especially in the context of the polydrug use patterns of most women — patterns that include the use of tobacco and alcohol, as well as the use of illegal drugs. The challenge is in trying to untangle the role of various substances in a child's development, while at the same time taking into consideration the impact of genetics and environment and how they relate to the histories of early deprivation and neglect found in many substance-exposed children.

Unfortunately, the best longitudinal studies of outcome present a bleak picture for alcohol-exposed children. Work by the clinical psychologist Ann Streissguth and her colleagues at the University of Washington School of Medicine examined a population of 415 adults and adolescents with prenatal alcohol exposure. The researchers found that over 90% of the subjects had mental health problems, over 60% had a disrupted school experience, 60% had trouble with the law, 50% had been confined in the criminal justice system, 49% had displayed inappropriate sexual behavior, and 35% had substance abuse problems. Studies such as this, however, are quite simplistic in structure, and, without underestimating their significance, it is important once again to keep in mind the old axiom: "Correlation is not causation." There are multiple factors that play into risk in a child's life, and most likely there were multiple opportunities for early intervention in the population under study that failed to materialize.

Still, these are the issues that are emerging as more and more alcohol- and drug-exposed children are reaching adolescence. Vulnerable to social pressure, unable to understand cause-and-effect actions, lacking the ability to express themselves, these children are set up in advance for the criminal justice system — a fact supported by national research, which reveals that the majority of individuals prenatally exposed to alcohol end up in jail. In Carlos's case, as in the case of many of the children with whom we work, the questions before the court are many: Did Carlos, despite his confession, really commit murder? Does Carlos comprehend the impact of his confession? Can Carlos, seeking social acceptance, understand the error he made in accepting the gun, or in telling police he shot the gun, though he knows he never fired it? Is Carlos fully able to participate in his defense? Should he really be charged as an adult? None of these is an easy question, and they remain with the court and the lawyers on each side to answer. However, Carlos's case brings forward even more important considerations for parents and professionals working with substance exposed children: Why wasn't Carlos identified earlier as being "at risk" because of his prenatal exposure and life circumstances? Could early intervention have prevented the sequence of events that led Carlos to the position he is in now, locked in juvenile detention and facing the prospect of life in prison? Just how much of his brain dysfunction is from his prenatal exposure and how much is from a life of neglect and emotional, sexual, and physical abuse?

Current research is looking at ways to answer some of these questions. Clearly, there are no simple solutions. But as we discuss the complex issues of behavior and risk in substance-exposed children, the core philosophy of the subsequent chapters will be based in the principle that prenatal alcohol and drug exposure must be understood in the context of damage to the child's brain. In this way, parents and professionals can be more readily available to the children, supporting them as they work through difficult issues. Approaches to discipline and management need to become less punitive and more thoughtful. With the right guidance, many children with prenatal exposure can learn to manage their own behaviors rather than relying wholly on external controls put in place by their parents or teachers or by social cues from unreliable peers.

From both a medical and a social standpoint, the bottom line is that prenatal exposure to alcohol or illicit drugs has tremendous implications for early intervention. Infants and toddlers with prenatal exposure often present early with difficulties that can be dismissed by the pediatrician or other professionals as a variant of normal: "She's just a fussy child." "Boys will be boys." But the child who is having difficulty with the usual tasks of infancy — feeding, sleeping, elimination — may be demonstrating one or more of a variety of brain-based disorders. Caregivers need to be aggressive in seeking help for their child, for the child's failure to receive appropriate interventions in the first two years of life can lead to further difficulties with emotional regulation and behavioral disorders as the child grows older. The "early" in early intervention is essential. A child learns and grows by building on milestones and skills. If initial or early skills are absent or late, the child cannot progress to the next developmental level; without intervention, the child is at great risk for escalating failures in all aspects of development. Early intervention is key to the child's reaching his or her full potential.

6   Off the Wall

When Brian awakens each dawn, he shrugs off the morning sun and rushes into the day, never satisfied to be in the present and always seeking something new. When he enters a room, he sucks up all available oxygen, talking at breakneck speed and overwhelming you with his busyness. Hands flying from his face, to a desk, to a hidden image on the wall that only he can see, his movement is non-stop.

Brian was born to a mother who used alcohol and cocaine heavily through pregnancy. He went home with her, but suffered severe abuse and neglect, so much so that by the age four he was placed in the custody of his grandfather. Soon after being named guardian, however, the grandfather was charged with child neglect because Brian had flung himself over a second story banister and suffered a mild concussion. Brian was referred to the Children's Research Triangle for an evaluation of the grandfather's ability to care for him.

It was immediately evident that there was no one who would have been able to manage Brian. With an IQ in the low 50s, Brian was in a state of constant movement. His fingers would reach for any object within arm's length, while his eyes darted from one target to the next. He literally banged into walls, his wild, hard-driving energy making it impossible for him to foresee what came next. Other children avoided his urgent hugs and tuned out his bursts of speech, but for adults who knew him Brian's personality and smile were an immediate draw.

Brian's case brings to mind a flight I took several years ago to a small community in Arkansas. I was settled comfortably in the narrow seat, tray table up, seat belt buckled, when our nine-seater prop plane suddenly lurched to the right. The pilot quickly recovered control, but my heart continued to race. I don't enjoy these little planes anyway, they make me uneasy, and unforeseen dips and bumps just add to my anxiety. The pilot's apology settled my nerves a bit, but it wasn't long until a bank of clouds moved in and began to play havoc with the plane. I dutifully tightened my seat belt and gripped the arm rests, suffering through the next ten minutes of foul weather.

During that time I felt completely out of control, unsure where the next bump or jolt would come from. All I could do was to hang on in terror as the plane dove and righted itself, rocking wildly from side to side and bouncing in the wind. When we finally burst through the clouds and emerged into the sunshine, my heart rate settled; I breathed easier. But that loss of control was frightening, an eerie reminder of what many substance-exposed children endure every moment of every day.

The brain basis of regulatory disorders

All children and adults need to feel in control. We have to know what to expect, be able to use information we need, and block out information we do not need to regulate ourselves in the context of our environment. On a daily basis, we block out extraneous stimuli, such as the buzz of an air conditioner or the whir of a fan. However, many substance-exposed children are unable to filter out unimportant stimuli. Lacking regulatory control, they easily become overwhelmed, appearing irritable and disorganized.

Regulatory control is accomplished through successful linking of information and environmental input to the prefrontal cortex, as mediated through the dopamine receptor system. If a child cannot move information into the prefrontal cortex to stimulate dopamine control, or if the dopamine receptor system is depleted, then the child cannot regulate his motor or behavioral response to the information.

Reviewing from chapter 3, cocaine is a good example of how drug use can interfere with the standard functioning of the dopamine receptor system. Cocaine blocks dopamine re-uptake in the proximal nerve ending, producing a "high" by increasing the amount of dopamine available at the nerve ends and increasing the excitation of the nerves. However, over a period of chronic exposure to cocaine, a dampening effect may be produced, depleting the dopamine receptors.

Nicotine has been shown to have a similar impact on the dopamine receptor system, and research data for many years have documented the increased rate of ADHD in children born to mothers who smoke tobacco during pregnancy. In the clinical population of children at Children's Research Triangle prenatally exposed to varying combinations of alcohol, drugs, and tobacco, 73% meet diagnostic criteria for ADHD. However, the children may not have classic ADHD based solely in genetics. Rather the ADHD may be based in depletion of the dopamine receptors due to the toxic effects of the children's prenatal exposure. Thus, many of these children respond positively to the use of stimulant medications.

Children exposed to alcohol present with a different neurological imprint. Alcohol's effect on the limbic system interferes with the transmission of information from its entry point in the brain to the prefrontal cortex. These children frequently have normal functioning dopamine levels, but, due to structural changes induced by alcohol exposure, the hippocampus, corpus callosum, or other areas of the limbic system simply cannot serve as the conduit for the information.

> It was one of those days in clinic when nothing seemed to be going right. Suzy, the last patient of the day, was no exception. "I give up," her adoptive mother said as she paced the clinic's interview room. "I can't do this

anymore." I was a bit surprised to hear the sound of defeat in her voice and asked what the problem was. "We adopted Suzy, she's our daughter, we love her, but I'm about to give her back to DCFS." The mom lowered herself into one of the two chairs in the room and took a breath. "Her pediatrician said she has ADHD and put her on Ritalin, but things just got worse. The last straw was a couple of weeks ago when we were playing in the front yard. All of a sudden Suzy darted toward the street! I yelled,'Suzy, stop, there's a truck coming!' Suzy stopped, looked at the truck, looked at me, and said,'I see it,' and just ran right into the street. The truck driver slammed on his brakes and barely missed her. I ran into the street and grabbed her, but it was just chaos! I can't do this anymore." I gave the mother a chance to calm herself, then turned to Suzy. "Suzy, you're nine years old. Didn't you see the truck coming?" Suzy peered up at me, her blue eyes squinting as she took time to choose her words. "I saw the truck coming. I just didn't think it would get there the same time I would."

Suzy is telling the truth; she saw the truck coming. However damage to the hippocampus, a part of the limbic system which links visual input in the occipital lobe to motor regulation in the prefrontal cortex, prevented her from recognizing it as a danger. With no thought of the consequences, she simply ran in front of a moving truck. Although Suzy does meet criteria for a diagnosis of ADHD, her decision to run in front of the truck did not come from "impulsivity" but from the inability to move information forward in the brain for a proper regulatory response from the dopamine receptor system. Placing a child like Suzy on Ritalin is like putting a child on speed; the Ritalin produces excess release of dopamine in a child who already has normal levels of dopamine functioning. Rather than stimulating the prefrontal cortex, the appropriate intervention for Suzy would focus on enhancing limbic system functioning by teaching Suzy ways to regulate her behavior.

Regulatory disorders

For many substance-exposed children, regulatory difficulties become evident early in infancy and in the toddler years. Infants and very young children with regulatory disorders have difficulties regulating their behavior, attention, motor, affect, and sensory processes; each of these areas of difficulty can occur alone or in combination. This makes it very hard for the infant to attain and remain in a calm and alert state and to exhibit a positive responsiveness to the caregiver. The infant's poorly organized response to external stimuli, such as bright lights or sound, or internal stimuli such as hunger or anger, can be shown in various ways—irregular breathing, startles, hiccups, and gagging. Commonly, parents who have an infant or a young child with regulatory problems worry about the child's sleeping and feeding difficulties and show concern that their baby or young child is fussy and irritable.

As the child moves into older infancy and the toddler years, regulatory difficulties appear in new ways. Gross motor disorganization becomes evident in erratic and uncoordinated movements and in constant movement patterns. Fine motor disorganization emerges as poor eye-hand coordination and jerky movements. Attentional disorganization manifests constant "driven" behavior, the inability to settle down, and perseveration (getting stuck) on small details. Babies with emotional disorganization appear sober or depressed, and have trouble calming themselves. Their range of emotions appears constricted, and they often exhibit abrupt shifts from being calm to crying inconsolably. To an outside observer, the toddler often is perceived as "spoiled" because of behaviors such as avoidance, negativity, being clingy and being demanding.

By the time the child reaches the preschool years, parents frequently describe the child as fearful or anxious. They express worry about their child's inability to play by himself or play well with other children. The child may be clumsy and uncoordinated, over- or under-responsive to sounds or speech, and limited in his attention span and ability to explain how he feels. He may lose his temper and have difficulty adapting to change. Teachers as well as parents often describe the child as very aggressive or hyperactive, and interpret these manifestations of dysregulation as willful "behavioral" problems on the part of the child.

In the end, what is most striking about children with regulatory disorders is the severely challenging ways the children tax their parents and other caregivers because of their unique sensory-processing patterns. When problems occur, the successful parent or caregiver needs to learn to identify the atypical demands of the young child and create an environment in which these demands can be met and worked through. Only when the child can attend to the external environment in a more functional way can the child's development get back on a typical course.

Attention-deficit / hyperactivity disorder

Attention-deficit/hyperactivity disorder (ADHD) is a good example of a regulatory disorder. Current research supports a model that explains ADHD as a failure to regulate activities that are under dopamine control. In addition, MRI and PET scan studies reveal that in children with classic, genetic ADHD, there is a loss of normal brain asymmetry as well as a reduction in the volumes of specific structures related to regulatory function. Lower blood flow in the prefrontal cortex, where dopamine resides, has been documented in children and adults with ADHD. These findings support the hypothesis that an underlying deficit in the dopamine system is a source of the behavioral difficulties in children with ADHD. It makes sense, then, that stimulant medications such as Ritalin that promote and enhance the transmission of dopamine are effective in the treatment of classic ADHD.

However, accurately understanding the child with symptoms consistent with a diagnosis of ADHD and deciding on appropriate treatment is complicated because there are four separate factors that make up attention: the ability to focus, to sustain, to encode, and to shift. Each of these functions is controlled by a different part of the brain. Assessment is further complicated because children at early school age are in the process of developing attention and concentration skills, as well as self-control. Even as they get older, children typically are active and interested in many different activities, and they may shift quickly between these different activities as their interest level fluctuates. Consequently, diagnosis becomes a challenge. Is the child demonstrating problems with attention because he is still mastering skills related to sustained attention and concentration, or, instead, because he is expressing the characteristic features of ADHD? The differentiation requires a broad and comprehensive evaluation of neuropsychological functioning.

It also is difficult to determine if prenatal substance exposure actually causes ADHD. Although ADHD is one of the most common diagnoses in children with a history of prenatal substance exposure, at least one longitudinal study of preschool children did not find evidence for a link between the exposure and decreased attentional abilities. Other studies corroborate these data, documenting a very small impact on sustained attention in four-year-olds. Consequently, it appears that prenatal substance exposure may not actually result in ADHD, per se. Instead, the difficulties may be based in other disorders including regulatory disorders, attachment disorders, anxiety problems, sensory integration deficits, and depression—all relatively common in children with prenatal exposure.

Putting hyperactivity into the context of regulatory disorders

Diagnostically, the difficulties we see in many young children who come to Children's Research Triangle for evaluation are best explained as a regulatory disorder, rather than within the framework of ADHD. Characteristics of regulatory disorder in young children include problems in regulating behavior, as well as in regulating physiological, sensory, attentional, motor, and affective processes. The children's difficulties are numerous:

- Motor disorganization
- Constant motion
- Over-reactivity to the sensation of movement
- Difficulty using visual-spatial cues
- Auditory processing problems
- Inability to settle down
- Difficulty modulating affect (moving rapidly from calm to screaming)
- Difficulty interacting with others (moving from avoidant to overly attached behaviors)
- Difficulty adapting to change
- Aggression
- Impulsivity
- Sleep disturbance
- Language processing problems
- Poorly differentiated fine motor activity

While this is a lengthy list, it is important to remember that all of these behaviors can derive from the same basic foundation: the children's difficulty processing the information and sensations they receive from internal and external sources. The importance of this approach to understanding hyperactivity is exemplified by the *motorically disorganized, impulsive* pattern, a regulatory disorder that can look quite similar to the classic picture of ADHD. Children in this diagnostic classification have a high activity level that is disorganized, impulsive, and often purposeless. In general, the children have a difficult time organizing themselves into a calm, positive state, particularly in the face of tension. This tension or arousal can be created by sensory stimulation or stress. When the children are in a situation in which they feel physiological and emotional stress, they tend to seek ways to reduce this stress level by discharging tension through disruptive behaviors. In this sense, the behaviors the children exhibit may not be adaptive, but they serve a purpose by helping the children regulate their stress and affect. Parents often articulate this well when they say that it feels as if their children need to get into a fight just to cry and release tension.

Children with a regulatory disorder also seek contact and stimulation through significant amounts of pressure, often achieved through unprovoked hitting, head banging, and other intrusions into people's physical space. Many of these sensation-seeking or excitable behaviors may be interpreted as aggression, though that is not typically the children's intent. Their under-reactivity to stimulation most likely results from their limited attention to regular sensory information (such as voices that are not raised). As we previously learned, this leads the children to seek out high levels of sensory input (e.g., turning lights on and off, hitting their head, and tearing up paper). Obviously, Ritalin will do nothing for these children and may in fact make things worse.

Executive functioning

Perhaps the best way to bring all this together is through the use of the umbrella term executive functioning first discussed in chapter 5. Executive functioning, which requires sensory integration and regulatory control, manages the interconnectivity of cognitive, behavioral, and emotional brain functions. Children with deficits in executive functioning abilities are not able to think ahead. This results in a variety of problems including the inability to self-direct behavior, maintain and integrate multiple bits of information, manage goals, stay on task, problem solve in a cognitively fluent manner, and place information into memory in order to complete a later task.

Executive functioning, put most simply, is the ability to plan and complete a task. It is a higher cognitive process that involves communication and organization across multiple brain sites and pathways. Because of the impact of prenatal exposure to alcohol, tobacco, and illicit drugs on these sites and pathways, the child is made very vulnerable to disorders of executive functioning. A child with such a disorder is not being disobedient by running out into the street. She simply has not made the connection between the words, "Do not run out into the street," and the literal motor action. Thus, she will need clear structure ("This is the boundary of our yard"), along with a physical barrier or marker as a cue in order to ensure her safety.

Executive functioning disorders can make it particularly difficult for children to perform operations that require attention, concentration, and mental control. Frequently children who have histories of prenatal alcohol exposure struggle to complete abstract processes, such as math problems, in their head. As another example, a child may know all his spelling words one day, yet be unable to spell a single word the next day. Although children often are accused of having "selective memory," in reality, the problem is not related to selection but to storage and retrieval. Because of the executive functioning disorder, the child is having difficulty recording information, storing it for later use, and then recalling that information. To remember her spelling words, the child will need special, often multisensory, cues.

Executive functioning deficits also may play an important role in social and learning difficulties. For instance, parents often say that prenatally exposed children have a hard time inhibiting their impulses and shifting between different activities. Routine transitions become difficult because the children have trouble moving from one activity to the next. This dynamic is especially evident in school, where changing from a reading lesson to a music lesson may set off tantrums and outbursts, particularly in the context of learning new information.

Prenatally exposed children often respond poorly to parents', teachers', or therapists' attempts to use behavior modification strategies to modify the child's behavior. Children with prenatal exposure have difficulties inhibiting previously learned responses; rather than adapting a new way of doing something, the children often repeat the same behaviors because they cannot use new skills to solve problems but simply revert back to prior knowledge. This often-inappropriate repetition can lead to a significant amount of frustration for parents and teachers, particularly when they do not understand the cause of the child's behaviors. Further behavioral difficulties grounded in executive functioning deficits often emerge because children with prenatal alcohol exposure appear to be unable to relate consequences to the misbehavior that caused them.

> Alex's adoptive mother, Carole, brought him into the clinic loaded down with reports from the school. Frustrated and angry with Alex and his teacher, she was ready to find blame. Carole handed over a one-inch stack of paperwork. "Here. I think it's time for medicine. By first grade, he should know how to behave!" In examining the reports, however, a clear pattern emerged. I turned to Alex. "What are the rules in the lunchroom?" Alex turned his round-cheeked face up to me and answered proudly, "You don't run, you don't pinch, you don't hit!" Carole sprang to her feet, vindicated. "See? He knows the rules. But look at the reports. He's constantly in trouble in the lunchroom. He just does this to spite the teacher and me! One of the school psychologists says he has oppositional defiant disorder and needs to go into a behavior disorder classroom."
>
> Carole clearly was overwhelmed by the pressure and negative reports from the school. Alex's birth mother used alcohol fairly heavily throughout early pregnancy. When she learned at about four months gestation that

she was pregnant, she stopped using. But in that first four months, damage was done to the corpus callosum, which showed on an MRI as significant thinning of its posterior portion. One of the two major functions of the corpus callosum is to transmit information between the two halves of the brain; however, when there is structural damage to the corpus callosum, this transmission is disrupted. Thus, Alex knows the rules cognitively; he just can't use the information to control his behavior. He does not have oppositional defiant disorder. He has structural damage to the corpus callosum, which prevents him from using information he recognizes at the cognitive level to guide and manage his behavior at the regulatory level.

All three children in this chapter meet criteria for a diagnosis of ADHD. However, meeting diagnostic criteria for ADHD does not necessarily indicate that the child should be treated with the same stimulant medications that are used for children with classic, genetic ADHD. In many cases, the executive functioning difficulties that make children look like they have ADHD result from regulatory disorders, sensory integration deficits, or both, and must be addressed accordingly. This is an important distinction that can only be made through appropriate neuropsychological testing of each child that includes assessment for regulatory disorders and sensory integration problems. This approach to evaluation will result in diagnostic conclusions that can direct an appropriate course of treatment. A child diagnosed with ADHD based on only behavioral observation will be placed immediately on medications. Treatment of a child with a regulatory disorder, on the other hand, will focus on a psychotherapeutic approach that addresses behavioral change through enhanced self-regulation.

7   Memory Becomes History

Bean sat silently. His mother, worn down by years of addiction and pain, gave a sigh. And sat. And didn't want to get up. "I can't," she breathed. "I can't understand him. He won't say a word to me." Tears welled in her eyes, streaking her heavy mascara and falling onto her working clothes—a dipping, plunge-necked blouse and faded jeans, two sizes too small. Bean sat silently. Elissa pursed her lips, as if trying to form words that had no shape. I had to ask my question carefully. "How long have you been clean?" She glanced up at me only briefly, sighed again, and tried to hold her voice steady, "A year." Bean didn't say a word.

The child was born in the midst of the cocaine epidemic of the mid-1980s. With no father as a namesake, the inspiration for Bean's name arose from the misreading of a liquor label. Working the streets as far into her pregnancy as she could, Elissa supported her habit by selling or trading her body, whichever opportunity arose. Avoiding doctors as long as she could for fear of giving herself away, Elissa showed up at the hospital in labor. One look at her track marks and inflamed nostrils, and the nurses ordered a toxicology screen. Of course it was positive, and Bean was born with high levels of cocaine in his system. Elissa was referred to a drug treatment program, went home from the hospital with Bean, and never looked back.

Elissa remembers Bean's early months well. "The shaking, that was the worst. He would look at me, and I knew it was my fault. I'd try to give him a bottle, but he'd shriek and cry and stiffen up and then he'd shake again. And all it did was make me want to go out and use." That was Bean's life over the first two years. Never abused but completely forsaken, left in a crib with a bottle propped on a pillow. By the time he was three, DCFS stepped in, and Bean began his journey through the child welfare system. He averaged one move every three months. No family could tolerate his aggressive and sexualized behaviors, his overactivity, or his foul mouth. "He's a bad influence, a child of the devil," one foster mother told me.

Either because Elissa had cleaned up her act or because DCFS simply had run out of options, five-year-old Bean was returned to his mother. Almost a year later, Elissa was trying her best to forge a relationship with Bean: a beautiful child, with dark hair, oval eyes, and olive skin that glistened in the light of the examining room. Physically, in the words of the DCFS caseworker, he was "perfect."

The first few months of their reunion were puzzling but happy ones. Elissa didn't mind that Bean had no words for her. She was more than willing to supply all the words that were needed; she had so much to say. But by nine months, Bean was becoming more difficult to be around and seemed to reject any of Elissa's efforts to comfort or love him. Her arms ached as she tried to fold him into her embrace and he would stiffen, arch his back, and throw his head as far away from her as possible. Her tears mingled with his as she grieved for her dashed expectations of motherhood.

History is a record of events. Memory is the perception of those events, the reconstruction of information gathered by the senses. Early in our lives we record events as they are perceived and store them in the deep recesses of memory. Years later those memories take on the structured shape of history as perceptions become truth, and the child's life evolves through his understanding of events as they occurred in the past. Core to this process is the young infant's perception of his primary relationship; it is within the context of this relationship through which the infant's emotional regulation, interpersonal relationships, and exploration of the environment unfold.

So when does memory begin? There is emerging evidence that a child's perception of his primary relationship may extend as far back as the womb. Studies of classical conditioning, habituation, and exposure learning reveal that the fetus does have a memory, which serves to support attachment to the mother, to promote breastfeeding, and, perhaps most interestingly, to encourage language acquisition. This suggests that the moment of birth is not the start of a baby's recollections but marks a transition from memory functioning in-utero to memory functioning ex-utero. For example, in a Northern Ireland study by the psychologist and fetal researcher Peter Hepper of Queen's University, Belfast, pregnant women watched the British television show *The Neighbors* an estimated 360 times throughout their pregnancy. Two to four days after birth, upon hearing the theme music to the show, their newborn infants became alert, stopped moving, and exhibited lower heart rates. The same babies showed no similar reaction to other, unfamiliar tunes, suggesting that their behavior was related to their remembering the theme song.

In another famous experiment by Anthony DeCasper and colleagues at the University of North Carolina, Greensboro, pregnant women read aloud Dr. Seuss's *The Cat in the Hat* at regular intervals throughout pregnancy. At birth the women's babies were hooked up to a variety of recordings they could select by sucking on a nipple at a particular rate of compression. After a few trials, the babies figured out what rate of sucking was needed to hear their mother's voice reading *The Cat in the Hat* and would preferentially suck at that speed. Studies exposing fetuses to various pieces of music or nursery rhymes have demonstrated similar findings of learned preferences.

Recently, it has been shown that fetal memory—the ability for the fetus to learn and preserve information from the mother's experiences—may be involved in a baby's preference for his mother's breast milk. A mother's diet flavors both the amniotic fluid and her breast milk. By swallowing amniotic fluid in-utero at twelve weeks gestation or later, the baby, once born, recognizes and prefers his own mother's breast milk, enhancing the baby's willingness to suck at the breast.

For years we have known that pregnant women grow an emotional attachment to their unborn child through the nine months of gestation. But is that emotional bond reciprocated by the fetus? Although more research needs to done before any hard conclusions can be drawn, there is a good deal of evidence that the fetus learns the speech characteristics of its mother prenatally and prefers its mother's voice to other female voices after birth. The mother's voice is a familiar stimulus in the baby's extra-uterine world. In addition to promoting responsiveness, it enables recognition of the mother as the primary object of attachment.

Unfortunately, negative prenatal experiences also can be stored in fetal memory. Frank Lake, a British psychiatrist who explored the effects of intrauterine life on later development, describes the fetus as being "marinated" in its mother's emotions. He postulates that the actual emotions of the mother-to-be can be transmitted to the fetus, especially during the first trimester. That view is supported in research such as experiments in Australia, which found that the fetus participated in the emotional distress of the pregnant mother as she watched a violent, twenty-minute segment of a Hollywood movie. Up to three months after birth, the infants showed recognition of the in-utero experience. In another study, newborn infants whose mothers had suffered depression during pregnancy displayed depression at birth in proportion to the mothers' depression scores. Maternal stress and anxiety also influence outcome at birth; high prenatal maternal anxiety levels have been linked with lower mental and motor development in the infant at eight months of age, lower mental development at two years, and higher levels of behavioral and emotional problems at six years of age. Longer-term studies are underway, but it appears that intrauterine sensory and emotional experiences could lay a powerful base for a child's developing mental health.

The chaos of memory

"What's your biggest concern?" I asked Elissa. "He won't talk to me, she answered. "He talks to everyone else, but he won't talk to me." Any further information I gathered from Elissa that first morning really didn't help. Bean went through a full evaluation at our clinic, and we enrolled Elissa and Bean in therapy with our mental health team. Over the next year, Elissa stayed the course, remained drug free, swore off the streets, and got her first job. Things were looking up.

But during the course of that year, Bean's therapist became concerned that Bean, at some point in the past, had been sexually abused. Bean's schoolwork was beginning to deteriorate, and his second grade special education teacher had reported repeated attempts of sexual aggression by Bean against other students. Elissa denied even the remote possibility of sexual abuse when Bean was in her care, and, believing her, we began to review records from his foster care settings. No clues emerged.

Months later, on one of those sunny January days in Chicago, Elissa again appeared at my door—this time unannounced. "I have to talk to you." I motioned her in, closed the door, and asked her what was wrong, trying to hide the rising anxiety I was feeling. She couldn't get the first word out. We both sat quietly, facing each other across the desk as she gazed down at the floor, her foot tracing the triangle of sunlight coming through the window. She took a breath and started again. "I did it." That's all she said. I wasn't sure what she meant.

"Did what?"

"I was scared, I was lonesome, I didn't have anyone else." The corner of her mouth was twitching. "I used Bean.

"It started when he was two months old. First I would just hold him against me . . . down there." Her eyes glanced downward quickly then came back to confront mine directly. "I would just hold him, but then I started rubbing him on me, and he would help me come, and then I would feed him. I figured he wouldn't know the difference and that he even liked it as much as I did. He didn't fight me at all and I knew I would stop as soon as he was old enough to know what I was doing but it just kept going and then when he was two he would start running away from me and now he won't talk to me."

An infant's sense of trust develops in the first years of life through interactions with a consistent and loving caregiver. All young children need a reciprocal relationship with at least one adult who is fully committed to the child; an adult who knows that child is the beginning and ending of all that is good. Without an early trusting relationship, the child's capacity for developing positive self-esteem and love for others cannot develop.

Infants who do not receive such love but instead suffer neglect, abuse, or unresponsiveness from their caregiver internalize this rejection as shame. Later in life this shame dominates the awareness of self. In Bean's case, the feeling of shame he has derived, not only from his mother's sexual abuse but also from the lack of a trusting relationship, continues to profoundly affect his life. Maladaptive development, as this process is called, evolves through successive failures of the young infant and maturing child to cope with the enlarging environment. Children go from maladaptation to a psychological disorder more rapidly when the early environment is one of physical and emotional abuse and neglect because no underlying sense of self, coping capacity, and resilience can develop.

Early childhood trauma

A century of study shows that traumatic memories in young infants generally remain unaffected by other life experiences. The memories may return at any time, with the same vividness as if the child were reliving the experience. In some ways this is counterintuitive, since prior to three years of age a child is preverbal and typically has no cognitive or narrative remembrance of a traumatic event. However, children do "remember" traumatic events through non-verbal, sensory recollection. Worse, such memories tend to resurface within a relational context, so that throughout life the individual's relationships are plagued by fear and anxiety.

Early childhood neglect can result in abnormal development of the brain, affecting some of the same areas of the brain as those disrupted by prenatal exposure to alcohol, tobacco, and illicit drugs. Neglect-induced abnormalities occur in brain systems that sense, perceive, process, interpret, and act on information withheld due to sensory deprivation. In studies of infants at risk, early childhood neglect is significantly associated with delayed cognitive development and reduced head circumference, independent of other risk factors. Interestingly, neglect, rather than abuse, is found to be the only type of maltreatment associated with cognitive delay.

Recent advances in neuroscience provide further insight into how childhood neglect may have an impact on early brain growth. While genetic factors regulate brain growth, sensory stimulation and experience are critical factors in final outcome. Animals reared in environments devoid of sight and sound tend to have small brains with reduced brain weight, length, and cortical depth. These changes correlate with a variety of changes at the cellular level, including fewer and smaller brain cells, decreased branching of the nerves, and reduced numbers of connections between the nerves.

Emotion is likely the primary avenue by which relationships and their meanings are organized within the brain. Early attachment relationships facilitate the growing child's capacity to organize emotions and adapt to future stressors. As a result, children with poor early attachment experiences have difficulty regulating their emotions and behaviors, especially when faced with stress. That is why sensory integration therapy has been found valuable in promoting an infant's emotional and behavioral regulation and enhancing the child's relationship with the primary caregiver.

The emotional development of a neglected child

Children who are severely neglected in their first two years of life may emerge with a set of peculiar behaviors, a condition called institutional autism. These children appear to be withdrawn, sullen, and resistant to touch. Repetitive behaviors such as head banging and rocking are common. If there is no loving and consistent caretaker to speak to the child or to engage in play, the deprived infant will not learn language skills at the appropriate time. Since language forms the basis for other cognitive functions, such as memory and goal-oriented behavior, a delay in language development restricts the child's all-around learning capacity.

Lack of early stimulation also may impede a child's capacity to decipher the meaning of non-verbal communication. Without the benefit of a loving adult to mirror the infant's expressions, the child may not be able to read the facial expressions and body gestures of others. Over time this may translate into poor or inappropriate social skills. In addition, children left unexposed to loving verbal interactions do not develop an understanding of cause-and-effect behavior: they may seem like they are tuning adults out, exercising defiance, or demonstrating deficits in attention.

Neglected infants who have spent their lives in drab surroundings that offer little variety of voice, music, color, or smell; scarce differentiation in the taste and texture of their food; or limited opportunity for movement, often lack the ability to deal with the outside world as they get older. Even after being removed from an environment of deprivation, a child's sensory systems remain poorly suited to process new experiences. Therefore, these children become over- or under-sensitive to stimuli around them, which contributes to emerging behavioral problems.

In fact, psychological effects of emotional trauma and the lack of a consistent attachment relationship may cause children to present a wide range of behavioral problems, especially in the realm of relationships. Although the child may be moved to a loving and stable adoptive home after a period of early neglect, she may be unable to utilize the stable and caring environment to develop a sense of security and to rely on her adoptive parents in an age-appropriate way. The previously neglected child may seem indifferent to her parents, insisting on doing things independently, and not even thinking of asking for help when the task is clearly beyond her capacity. She may shy away from comfort when distressed, or, alternatively, may seek out someone other than the parent for affection. Interestingly, children with a history of early neglect often are indiscriminately friendly, showing no initial cautiousness with unfamiliar people and preferring the presence of strangers to those they know.

Attachment disturbances

Unfortunately, many substance-exposed children have early histories devoid of attachment experiences that ensure healthy growth and development. Without the presence of an attuned caregiver who responds to needs as they emerge and provides stimulating and comforting interactions, the children may suffer feelings of displacement and loss. In addition, they may lack a feeling of safety and security and have difficulty trusting others in relationships. Because adults in their lives have so often proven unpredictable, undependable, or even abusive, neglected children feel extremely vulnerable and threatened by closeness or intimacy. They are afraid to open up to adults. This distrust is a cornerstone of attachment disturbances. Even in the absence of neglectful or abusive caregivers, neglected and abused children will continue to respond to caregivers based upon expectations of maltreatment. Efforts made by foster or adoptive parents to provide security or nurturance, despite being well intentioned, may be refused by the child with attachment disturbances, as recollections of previous abuse can bring forth fear and anxiety. Instead of embracing the affection of new parents, the children often demonstrate bizarre or unpredictable behavior aimed at restoring feelings of control. The children's inability to securely attach to a reliable, supportive caregiver presents great challenges later in their development, because it is through successful relationships with others that children gain a healthy, positive picture of themselves.

Posttraumatic stress disorder

Children who have been physically or sexually abused, or severely neglected, may demonstrate symptoms of complex posttraumatic stress disorder (PTSD) years after the trauma. The most obvious behaviors are related to the child's poor emotional affect and an inability to control impulses. The child suffers a damaged perception of himself, with a sense of being different or ineffective. He may seem to "space out" and will describe a sensation of leaving his body. Interpersonal relationships may be characterized by extremes: either mistrusting adults or being extremely dependent on adults. Ironically, the child's perception of the perpetrator of early trauma often is idealized and distorted, with no basis in reality. Frequent bodily complaints, feelings of hopelessness, fear and anxiety, sleep problems, nightmares, and trouble with attention and focus are common symptoms. These may be punctuated by flashback episodes and reactions to triggers that serve as reminders of the early experiences. Because the obvious behaviors and signs of emotional distress can be so diffuse, children often receive mistaken diagnoses of ADHD or depression, and are given the wrong medications to treat their symptoms.

Co-occurring mental health disorders in substance-exposed children

It is important to address issues of early attachment, relationships, and mental health not only because so many children with prenatal exposure have suffered significant neglect and trauma in early childhood, but also because many of them have been wards of the child welfare system.

Foster care is a risky venture for any child. Large studies have shown that about half of foster children from two to fourteen years of age have clinically significant emotional or behavioral problems. Adolescents in foster care are much more likely to experience depression, anxiety, loss of behavioral or emotional control, and poor overall psychological well-being as compared to youth in the general population. For example, one study in Great Britain that followed up children's mental health after thirty years found that adults with a history of having been in foster care were more likely to have a psychiatric illness than matched adults who had grown up in their biological home.

Arguably, the most impressive study of the impact of early psychological trauma comes from Kaiser Permanente Health Care, a managed care system in California. As a closed system of care, physicians at Kaiser are able to follow their patients from cradle to grave, allowing for the collection of valuable longitudinal data. In this study, Kaiser's research team found that recurrent and severe emotional or physical abuse, sexual abuse involving physical contact, or being raised in a household with an alcohol or drug user had a profound effect fifty years later. Children living with a family member imprisoned, mental illness in the household, or without either biological parent present in the home also showed these effects. Among children living in any of these conditions, negative psychosocial experiences were likely to transform into organic diseases such as diabetes, high blood pressure, and heart problems, or emerge as social malfunction and mental illness.

Granted, there are factors that can mediate the impact of early trauma. Was the trauma isolated or ongoing? Was the perpetrator a stranger or a family member? What was the frequency and intensity of the trauma and at what point in the child's development did it occur? What is the child's level of cognitive functioning, his disposition, his temperament? Has there subsequently been an attuned, consistent attachment figure that has served as a safe haven for the child?

The importance of these issues becomes clear as we begin to look at the "secondary disabilities" described among adults who have had a history of prenatal alcohol exposure. Numerous studies of children from 5 to 13 years of age have documented high rates of mood disorders, disruptive behaviors, antisocial behaviors, ADHD, depressive disorders, oppositional defiant disorder, conduct disorder (CD), and specific phobias. Many times children have more than one mental health diagnosis, making it harder for them to succeed in school. When children internalize difficulties experienced in the classroom, they may feel they are failures or come to believe they are simply "bad." Often what emerges is a vicious downward cycle of poor performance and depression.

Although it is clear that there is an increased rate of psychopathology in children with prenatal exposure to alcohol and illicit drugs, the question remains as to how much of the high prevalence can be attributed to the biologic effects of prenatal exposure, how much is due to genetic propensity, and how much can be traced back to environmental trauma. At Children's Research Triangle, we attempted to evaluate the relative impact of biological vs. environmental effect through a study of 119 foster and adopted children, 63 of whom had been prenatally exposed to alcohol and illicit drugs and 56 of whom had not been exposed to any substances (Table 7.1).

Diagnosis	Prenatally Exposed N = 63	Non-exposed N = 56	General Population
TABLE 7.1 MENTAL HEALTH DISORDERS IN SUBSTANCE-EXPOSED AND NON-EXPOSED CHILDREN FROM THE CHILD WELFARE SYSTEM AS COMPARED TO A NATIONAL POPULATION			
ADHD	75%	54%	7%
Anxiety Disorder	8%	11%	4%
Attachment Disorder	11%	14%	< 1%
Disruptive Behavior Disorder	6%	16%	2%
Elimination Disorder	16%	5%	3%
Mood Disorder	19%	38%	2%
PTSD	19%	27%	5%

Both groups of children had significantly higher rates of mental health disorders than found in the general population of children as documented through a variety of national studies. Of interest, although ADHD occurs at a rate many times higher in both the substance-exposed and non-exposed children than in the general population, there is a statistically significant higher rate of ADHD among the substance-exposed children than the non-exposed children. This finding is consistent with the earlier discussion of the impact of exposure to alcohol, tobacco, and illicit drugs on fetal brain development. However, the elevated rates of the other mental health disorders were essentially the same in the two groups of children from the child welfare system, except for mood disorders, which occurred more commonly among the non-exposed children.

To explore these issues further, our research team set up a series of statistical equations that examined the relative impact of specific biological factors (i.e., growth failure, poor brain growth, the presence of facial features associated with FAS) and environmental factors associated with placement in the child welfare system (i.e., length of time in the current placement, number of placements prior to the current home, and the occurrence of physical abuse and neglect). Our analyses revealed that the number of placements in the child welfare system played the most significant role in putting both substance-exposed and non-exposed children at risk for mental health disorders, while prenatal exposure had only a distant secondary role. These findings are in line with those of Susanne Fryer and colleagues at San Diego State University's Center for Behavioral Teratology, who also showed that higher rates of psychopathological conditions among alcohol-exposed children were associated with placement in a foster or adoptive home. The bottom line, of course, is that it is most likely a combination of prenatal and postnatal factors that contributes to the high rates of mental health disorders we find in alcohol-exposed populations.

Clearly, more research is necessary. But the fact that environmental trauma plays such an important role in placing substance-exposed children at risk for severe mental health problems is not surprising. Biological changes in the brain induced by prenatal alcohol and drug exposure result in behavioral problems that set up the child for a series of placement failures in foster or adoptive homes. As a rule, each time the child is moved to a new home, behavior becomes worse, and the new family is even more likely to disrupt the placement. The cumulative effect of these aborted placements is a cycle of deterioration and increasing chaos in the child's life. The implications are profound: we are taking biologically vulnerable children and placing them in a child welfare system that preys on their vulnerability.

> I last saw Bean when he was fourteen years old. He was leaving Chicago, destined for California, and had come to tell me goodbye. His face still held the charm of his childhood, but there was a hypervigilance to his eyes hardened by the life he had been born into. His anger lent a sharp edge to his words; gang tattoos covered his arms. He wasn't using drugs — he had seen what they had done to his mother. But he sold them, earning his name on the streets and claiming his ascendancy into the safe haven of his gang "brothers." He talked about his mother's

whoring, her continuing drug use, his intermittent stays in group homes, and his failure in almost every aspect of his life. No amount of therapy could resolve the confusing and conflicted feelings of love, fear, and abhorrence he had for his mother. He was a young man who I felt deserved an apology from the world for the way his life had unfolded.

I ask you to think of Bean—prenatally exposed to alcohol and cocaine, sexually abused by his mother, shuffled from home to home in the child welfare system, reunited with his perpetrator for whom he holds intense and conflicting feelings of love, fear, revulsion, and anger. Placing Bean on medication may follow as the clinician's instinctive response, but this is not the "fix" for Bean; nor is this the solution for most children in the child welfare system. What needs to be done, instead, is to provide support to the foster and adoptive families that bring these children into their homes. By preparing families to manage the child's difficult behaviors and address the child's mental health problems, we lessen the likelihood of a disrupted placement.

As parents and clinicians, we cannot absolve children of their negative memories, but we can cultivate emotional bonds that open the child's reservoir of hidden strengths. When the relationship between the child and the family blossoms, the specific facts of the child's story recede in importance as new memories and history take precedence. It is a mistake to focus on "behavior management" alone, for this ignores the mental health basis of many behavioral difficulties seen in substance-exposed children. Only through thorough evaluation and concentrated attempts to integrate behavioral and therapeutic interventions, can we look beyond the behavior we see to understand the source of that behavior. This is how we can make a difference in the ultimate history of the child.

PART II
THE CONTEXT OF NORMAL

8 The Developmental Nature of Behavior

It was a hot summer afternoon in Chicago, and I was driving to the local swimming pool with my two seven-year-old granddaughters. They were spending their annual summer week with us, and every day was a new adventure as I fine-tuned parenting skills I had long ago put aside when my own children had themselves reached the point of parenting. On the way to the pool, I was trying to fulfill a promise I had made to my daughter-in-law. Earlier in the week, when she and my son had left the girls in our care, she had been very clear in her request: "They need to get their hair cut. Can you take them sometime this week?" Obviously, I had waited until the last minute, but I had thought we would blow through this task with no problems, making it to the swimming pool as it opened for the afternoon.

Things went as planned with Stav. Anxious to get to the pool, she allowed the shampoo and cut, with only a hint of a scowl. However when I moved to Noam, I was met with crossed arms, a defiant deeply lined forehead, hard set eyes, and a firm, "No." I was taken aback, but I summoned my best parenting techniques and approached her with what I thought was an appropriate mix of concern and firmness. It didn't work. After three minutes of conversation descended into cajoling and bribery, I gave up. That, after all, is the privilege of grandparenting—it's really not my problem. She was heading home in two days, and her mother could deal with the out-of-control hair. We headed to the pool and had a great time.

I tell this story because the very next Monday, I had a new family come into the clinic and recite an almost identical story involving their eight-year-old son. The only difference was that he had been adopted in infancy from a mother who had used alcohol and cocaine throughout pregnancy. I gathered the history, listened to all the behavioral difficulties the parents recited, and examined the child. Diagnosis? Normal kid. Despite being labeled as a "high risk" child and having acquired previous diagnoses of oppositional defiant disorder and conduct disorder, this was a normal eight-year-old boy. Granted, there were some issues to deal with, but the reality is sometimes a kid is just a kid. The parents at first greeted my clinical pronouncement of "normal kid" with an air of skepticism, but they adjusted quickly. Over the past year, with minor changes in parenting style and approach, he's been doing fine.

Admit it, we've all been there: caught in an escalating struggle with a child as he falls apart before our eyes. We feel helpless and isolated as we lose control of the situation. If it's a public setting, we feel others' eyes on us, judging our apparent incompetence with subtle expressions of disapproval. Children can be trying, even in the best of circumstances; and when those difficult standoffs occur, the first question parents of substance-exposed children often ask is "Is this because of the drugs, or is this normal?" Unfortunately, sometimes our pre-conceived notions of "risk" get in the way of really understanding the child and his behavior.

As one might imagine, behaviors, both acceptable and unacceptable, change over time. When children become older, their behavior becomes more focused and specific, with increasing self-control and responsibility. The exploratory behavior of toddlers gradually gives way to behavior that is purposeful and organized.

By the time children enter school, they show the beginning of industriousness and initiative.

It is not difficult to fathom how a behavior considered normal at one age can be a problem at another. A good example is separation anxiety. In the first and second years of life, it is very normal for children to show anxiety and fear about being separated from their parents. As children mature, this anxiety typically decreases until the behavior occurs only in a handful of situations. Many children become upset about leaving their parent on the first day of kindergarten, but in general this anxiety subsides as the child becomes comfortable in the new surroundings. If the behavior continues throughout the primary grades, however, it is not normal. Now it constitutes a legitimate problem

Development often is conceptualized as occurring along trajectories, or pathways. A child's development occurs along multiple trajectories simultaneously, with each trajectory signifying a different domain or area of development, including cognitive, emotional, social, interpersonal, and motor. Often a child may be on a healthy trajectory in one domain but on a less than optimal trajectory in another. These trajectories are assumed to be linear and continuous, unless something occurs to redirect the pathway. Thus, the goal for parents and those who work with children is to affect the trajectory in a positive way, so less optimal pathways are impeded and the child's long-term trajectory is modified in a normal and healthy direction.

When behavioral problems occur, there is a tendency to forget that at times the child is "just being a kid." The parent or teacher should not assume that every inappropriate behavior or series of behaviors indicates the presence of a problem. Often, even the child who has been identified as having behavioral problems may simply be exhibiting behavior typical of children of the same age. All children, at different times, may exhibit a degree of inattention, distractibility, withdrawal, aggressiveness, mild disobedience, and off-task behavior.

Beyond "normal": When behaviors become problems

Those who live and work with children often ask how to know when a behavior is "abnormal" or problematic versus when it is merely a variation within a wide range of "normal." There are four essential criteria for making this determination: frequency of the behavior, duration of the problem, whether the behavior is having a detrimental impact on the child's learning, and whether the child's relationship with peers or adults is negatively affected.

Frequency refers to how often a behavior occurs and whether it occurs often enough to have an impact on a child's success in one of the domains of development. Recording how often a child fails to complete assignments at school, the number of times a child jumps up from his seat at the dinner table, or the rate at which a child interrupts others in conversation can help answer the critical question: "Do these behaviors occur with such frequency that they interfere with healthy learning or relationships?"

Duration refers to how long a behavior persists. If an undesired or inappropriate behavior persists for so long that the child's performance or social interactions are affected, then the behavior becomes problematic. To measure duration, a caregiver might assess how long a child remains off task or how often a child withdraws from social situations.

In most cases, simultaneous assessment of frequency and duration is the key first step in determining if substance exposure has had a harmful effect on the child's development. For example, the child may be off task for several minutes at a time (duration), while making distracting noises or getting out of his chair several times during the same class period at school (frequency). It may be necessary to consider both the time off task as well as the frequency of other negative behaviors that occur during that time. However, the most important consideration is whether the behavior is having an adverse impact on the child's learning, social relationships with peers, or interactions with adults.

Types of children's behavioral problems

On observing a child's behaviors, a pattern of aggressiveness, withdrawal, unhappiness, anxiety, or other difficulties may emerge. However, many times the behaviors do not appear to have a pattern or to be caused by identifiable events. For example, a child may suddenly become aggressive for no apparent reason, leading to confusion and uncertainty on the part of the caregiver as to how to intervene. Having a systematic understanding of children's behavioral problems is important if you are to develop effective interventions for your child.

Over-controlled behavior

Over-controlled behavior (Table 8.1) refers to a behavioral pattern in which children expend much energy controlling their feelings and inhibiting their behavior. These children often exhibit withdrawal and social isolation and may be difficult to identify because they do not disrupt the classroom or family. Such children sit in the back of the classroom and are perceived as being shy, compliant, and reluctant to engage in activities.

TABLE 8.1 OVER-CONTROLLED BEHAVIOR
• Secretiveness
• Worry
• Lack of communication
• Complaints of being unloved
• Fearfulness
• Staring
• Withdrawal
• Sulking
• Peer difficulties
• Obsession with perfection

Over-controlled behaviors sometimes are referred to as "internalizing patterns." The child's feelings are directed inwardly so that the child experiences depression, anxiety, or low self-esteem and lacks self-confidence and feelings of efficacy. The parent and classroom teacher should be alert to indications of these patterns, as most children with these types of problems are never identified.

CASE STUDY: **Susie — talkative**

Susie is talking in class without permission, and the teacher reprimands her. Susie becomes very quiet for the next hour. However, the adult supervisor observing her on the playground during recess reports that Susie interacts well and shows no signs of withdrawal. Back in the classroom, she behaves appropriately, responds well to directions, and completes tasks.

Case Discussion

Since past observations of Susie's behavior suggest that usually she is well behaved, her brief withdrawal behavior in response to the reprimand is situation-specific and should not be considered an internalizing pattern. Almost all children will talk out of turn like Susie at times (i.e., "just being a kid"), so hers is not a serious problem that warrants specific interventions.

CASE STUDY: **Sammy — withdrawn**

Sammy does not seem to enjoy working with other children but spends much of his time alone, both in and out of the classroom, and rarely smiles. He has a need for everything to be perfect, and lack of perfection seems to confirm his own beliefs of his inadequacy. He rarely participates in classroom activities or volunteers answers. He seems very tense and uncomfortable when called upon to participate, often lowering his eyes and not responding. When he does respond he frequently speaks so softly he cannot be heard.

Case Discussion

Although much more information would be needed to make a formal diagnosis, the withdrawal described here is part of a chronic pattern that is interfering with Sammy's schoolwork. Children with a low tolerance for frustration frequently withdraw from stressful or challenging situations. Fear and insecurity often prompt this behavior, with the child lapsing into daydreaming as an escape from anxieties.

The essential difference between Susie and Sammy is that Susie's behavior is in direct response to a specific situation and not characteristic of a chronic pattern, whereas Sammy has exhibited a long-term pattern of dysfunction which seems to bridge different situations and conditions.

CASE STUDY: **Brian — withdrawn**

Brian is a very quiet first-grader who spends most of his time alone. He does not join group activities and stands on the edge of the playground watching other children play. In the classroom he quietly sits at his desk, often sucking his thumb and gazing into space. He has never brought in items for show-and-tell and does not volunteer any answers or participate in class discussions.

Case Discussion

Brian is an example of an internalized/withdrawn child who is likely quite shy. He appears to be unhappy and detached. He is withdrawn from others and has very few friends. Children like Brian may not be identified as a problem because they are compliant and cooperative in the classroom and at home. These children frequently withdraw or lapse into daydreaming as an attempt to escape anxiety. As a result of failure or mistreatment, they often have a poor self-image and negative expectations of themselves and others.

CASE STUDY: **Yolanda — defeatist**

Yolanda is of average ability but appears to put forth very little effort to do her homework. She complains that assignments are too hard before even attempting them. When her mother gives her individual attention, she finds Yolanda is very capable of doing the work assigned. But Yolanda gets frustrated and disgusted very easily; instead of trying to solve a problem she gives up, convincing herself she cannot handle it and calling herself "stupid."

Case Discussion

Yolanda tends to internalize her feelings of anger and helplessness, setting up a pattern of failure that serves to reconfirm her beliefs. She has a low self-image and is defeated before she even starts a task. When she begins a project she applies very little effort, giving up as soon as she encounters any difficulty.

Under-controlled behavior

Under-controlled behavior (Table 8.2) patterns are more easily identified in children than over-controlled patterns because the behavior that emerges tends to be disruptive. "Acting out" is one way that these types of behaviors are labeled. While children with over-controlled behavior tend to turn their feelings inward, the under-controlled ("externalizing") child has difficulty inhibiting or controlling behavior and expresses his feelings outwardly, usually against others.

TABLE 8.2 UNDER-CONTROLLED BEHAVIORS	
Aggressive Type	• Inability to sit still • Overactivity • Failure to complete tasks • Difficulty following directions • Inattentiveness • Impulsive behavior • Stealing
Overactive Type	• Defiance • Oppositionality • Aggressiveness • Fighting • Refusal to follow directions • Class disruptions • Temper tantrums • Impulsive behavior • Stealing • Destructiveness

There are two categories of under-controlled behaviors. Children with a conduct disorder or oppositional defiant disorder are ordinarily categorized as "aggressive" because they have difficulty managing aggression and anger. The second category of children is those who meet criteria for ADHD. These children have difficulty sustaining attention to tasks and are distractible and impulsive. Sometimes they are overactive or hyper. Their difficulty with self-management may or may not include problems with aggression.

Children who exhibit these types of behaviors are likely to be difficult and disrupt the family and the classroom. While some children exhibit a range of behavior that applies to both the overactive and aggressive categories, other children fall exclusively into one category. It is important to distinguish children who have difficulty with attention and distractibility but nonetheless are able to control their aggression and anger, from those who cannot manage their behavior — and vice versa. Strategies for addressing these different behavioral patterns are distinct, and thus the behaviors need to be carefully assessed.

CASE STUDY: Enrico — aggressive / oppositional

Enrico has a history of becoming aggressive and defiant when given directions and sometimes openly refuses to do as he is asked, directing hostility toward his mother. If his brother teases him, Enrico becomes very angry and responds with aggression, sometimes hitting or kicking his brother. These incidents usually occur while playing outdoors, but also have been reported at school. Although this behavior does not occur every day, it happens with enough frequency (two to three times per week) and is sufficiently disruptive that his mother cannot ignore the problem. Enrico has few friends and hangs out at school with other students who have a tendency to get into trouble with teachers and administrators.

Case Discussion

Enrico is demonstrating under-controlled or "externalized" aggressive behavior that is a problem at home and in the classroom and relegates him to a peer group that serves to reinforce his behavior. For many oppositional children, defiance to authority is an effort to maintain a sense of personal control in situations in which they feel vulnerable. This can reflect negative experiences with parents who have not provided the child with enough sense of control or who have responded punitively to the child's attempts to seek independence. Under-controlled children often have difficulty sharing with other children as they feel the need to control situations in which their power is at risk of being stolen. Because of underlying insecurity, such children also are very sensitive to name calling and other small slights.

CASE STUDY: Andrea — distractible / impulsive

Andrea tends to be very distractible in class. Whenever multiple activities are occurring at the same time or someone new walks into the room, she loses track of what she is doing. This often results in her not completing tasks or assignments. In addition, she is impulsive, jumping to quick, incorrect responses on written materials, even though she knows the right answer when offered one-on-one help. Usually when working on assignments, she completes only about half of the work before getting lost or disorganized. She has few friends because they tire of her apparent immaturity and constant disruptive behavior.

Case Discussion

Andrea is demonstrating under-controlled behaviors typical of attention-deficit disorder (ADD)/ADHD patterns. She is disruptive in the classroom because she has difficulty managing her behavior well enough to function academically and socially. ADD/ADHD experts believe these problems are a result of a hereditary biochemical brain disorder that is based in abnormalities of the dopamine receptor system. In addition to a genetic basis for ADD/ADHD, recent research discussed in previous chapters shows that brain damage from prenatal alcohol or illicit drug exposure during pregnancy can produce behaviors that are consistent with a diagnosis of ADD/ADHD.

CASE STUDY: **Martin — aggressive / impulsive**

Martin is eating dinner with the family. His brother accidentally brushes by Martin as he sits at the table, causing Martin's napkin to fall on the floor. Martin jumps out of his seat and pushes his brother to the floor. Martin also displays this behavior frequently on the school playground and during group work.

Case Discussion

Martin's reaction represents typical aggressive/impulsive patterns of behavior. Recent literature indicates that hostile aggressive behavior often is a result of modeling by parents who use excessive physical punishment as a means of discipline. Thus, rather than teaching skills of conflict resolution, social problem solving, self-management, and communicative techniques to help the child define and verbalize feelings, punitive parents teach their children that "a good offense is the best defense." Such children often respond to even small slights as if they were threats to their safety. A tendency for the child to exhibit overall impulsive behavior and a low threshold for frustration contribute further to the aggressive responses Martin displays.

Mixed behavior

Many children show signs of both internalizing and externalizing behaviors. We refer to these patterns as "mixed," that is, those that are not clearly of *only* the under-controlled or over-controlled type. Because under-controlled behavior patterns are, by definition, disruptive in nature, they may overshadow over-controlled patterns. Thus, it should not be assumed that internalizing problems do not exist just because a child displays only under-controlled patterns. Parents and teachers trying to intervene with a child will be most successful if they first determine what behavioral pattern is most characteristic of the child and is driving the observable behaviors.

Case Study: **Bobby — withdrawn / socially isolated**

Bobby is a quiet, shy seven-year-old boy with few friends. Bobby's foster brothers and many of his peers tease him and call him names. At home Bobby spends most of his time alone. At school, when the class is divided into groups to work on a project, members of Bobby's group have been heard making unkind remarks loud enough for everyone in the class to hear. Both at home and at school, Bobby is provoked and becomes aggressive toward others. Although the behavior is usually brief, it adds to his difficulties, magnifying his sense of isolation and detachment.

Case Discussion

In this situation, Bobby shows both under-controlled and over-controlled problems, although withdrawal and social isolation predominate. Establishing a "we" feeling and positive group identity, whether at home or at school, is the best solution for peer rejection problems. Teaching Bobby pro-social values such as self-control, self-discipline, and the need to care for oneself, will minimize the frequency at which he experiences peer rejection problems.

Children with mixed behaviors can be confusing. In addition to problems with distractibility and impulsive behavior, these children may have difficulty managing their anger and may frequently experience high levels of anxiety and feelings of depression. Thus, as we view a child and his behavioral difficulties, we must individualize our conceptual approach to understand the child's behavior.

Case Study: **Nilda — distractible**

Nilda never seems to finish an assignment. She cannot stay in her seat. She is constantly getting up to wander into the hall or go over to the window to see what is going on. She almost never gets back on task after a distraction.

Case Discussion

Nilda's is an example of under-controlled/attention-deficit behavior. She is easily distracted and unable to sit still and complete tasks—behaviors characteristic of children with ADD. Research has found that teaching children to self-monitor their behavior has been very successful in helping students remain on task; many children with such difficulties simply are unaware of the frequency at which they tune out. However, this type of direct cognitive intervention will not work with younger school-age children. At this age, environmental approaches to block out distractions such as providing a study area at home or a study carrel at school, monitoring the child's schoolwork, and giving the child headphones to play white noise or soft music will be more beneficial.

CASE STUDY: **Lucy — controlling**

Lucy has outbursts of anger when her requests are not immediately met. When reprimanded by the teacher she becomes sullen and pouts, or tries to lay blame on someone else. She asks for help, but when the teacher tries to explain the assignment she hums, stares out the window, or taps her pencil repetitively on the desk. In group situations she is very controlling. If she cannot be the "leader" the entire time she refuses to participate and withdraws from the group. She always is the last to get in line for lunch and for recess and often pretends not to hear instructions even when they are directed specifically at her.

Case Discussion

Lucy's behavior is referred to as "mixed" because her behavior is not clearly internalizing or externalizing; however, the common thread within her behavior pattern is her desire to seek control. A child living in a home that is in constant conflict lives in a world that is unreliable and unpredictable. As a result, the child is confused as to how to please her parents and how to respond to social situations appropriately. Often these children try to establish a sense of control over their lives by resisting external controls. Techniques that encourage children to express their feelings directly, however, will counteract that tendency, allowing the child to talk through her sense of vulnerability. By giving their child choices and options, parents and teachers can strengthen the child's confidence that she has a role in deciding what she does, giving her a greater sense of control over her life.

9 Sources of Child Behavior Problems

It is common for parents and teachers to ask why children exhibit particular behavioral and emotional difficulties. Understandably, these adults believe that knowing the causes will help them develop methods to deal with the problems. It also is common for adults to assume behavioral issues are the product of some inherent characteristics of the child. However, viewing the child as the sole or primary source of behavioral problems is inappropriate. Instead, we need to consider multiple sources of influence including ecological factors, child-specific characteristics, and interactions between these two.

Ecological factors

Ecological factors are characteristics of a child's home, family relationships, neighborhood, and school climate that influence the child's development and well-being. It is important to remember that each child is embedded within a complex matrix of ecological factors and that the influences may be indirect and difficult to discern. Children, for instance, are affected by the behavior of their parents, but their parents are affected by the neighborhood environment, economic stress, and other environmental conditions in which they live. The larger school environment in which a classroom is situated affects the child directly, but also affects the child indirectly through how the larger environment influences the teacher and other school personnel who work with the child. Inevitably, children will bring the influence of the larger ecologies to the home and classroom in ways that can contribute to behavior, learning, and relationship problems.

Home and family relationships

Ineffective parenting, including difficulty setting limits or use of inappropriate punishment, can affect a child's behavior as well as her response to authority. If violence permeates the family's life, the home environment likely is unpredictable and lacks structure. In addition, families may be struggling to manage the larger ecological conditions associated with poverty, unsafe neighborhoods, lack of community resources, poor medical care, and concerns about meeting the family's basic needs. All of these conditions can contribute to disorganization in the child's life and escalate behavioral regulation problems.

Classroom factors

Adults often attribute the source of behavioral problems to either the child or home, but there is ample evidence to indicate classroom ecological factors contribute significantly. Consideration of the classroom environment is thus critical for the successful management of behavioral problems, for it is much easier to change the circumstances that contribute to a problem than it is to change the child's behavioral characteristics. If a child has an attention problem, for instance, that is intensified in situations in which there are multiple distractions—it will be far more effective to alter or remove the provocation than to train the child to be more attentive. Although the child still may have the attention problem, it will be much less apparent.

Many types of classroom situational factors can influence a child's behavior and become the focus for intervention in the classroom:

- Large class sizes or grouping problems
- Structure or arrangement of the classroom
- Unrealistic, unclear, or inappropriate expectations from adults
- Tasks or instructional conditions that are inappropriate for the child
- Presence of several children who present management difficulties
- Lack of administrative and instructional support for the teacher

Because of its prevalence one of these situational factors—unrealistic expectations from adults—merits further discussion. If a child is expected to do more than he can do, he may become frustrated. Despite his parent's best hopes, no amount of coaxing, coercion, or behavior management will enable him to do something he cannot do. A child may react negatively to the pressure by refusing to cooperate or by exhibiting disruptive behavior, inattentiveness, or inconsistent performance. When adults are unaware a child is being asked to do something beyond his ability, they may incorrectly assume that the behavior is a sign of willful disobedience. We will address the difference between skill and performance deficits later, but for now suffice it to say that a simple change in expectations often will solve the problem.

Child-specific factors

Child-specific factors describe a broad range of circumstances that increase a child's vulnerability to the development of behavioral problems. Often enhanced by home and family difficulties, they include several subgroups:

- Neurological/biological factors
- Developmental problems

- Emotional factors
- Motivational factors

Neurological/biological factors

Biological factors generally are present when a child has a history of a medical or physical problem that has accompanying behavioral manifestations such as attention difficulties, impulsive behavior, or low tolerance for frustration. As we have discussed in previous chapters, because of the structural and functional damage to the fetal brain that may be induced by prenatal substance exposure, children who are prenatally exposed often have difficulty regulating their behavior and easily reach a level of overstimulation. Rarely are they able to regain control of their behavior once that threshold is surpassed. The same can be said of children exposed to violence in the home or children who have suffered early emotional or physical trauma.

Some professionals who work with children assume that if behavioral problems have a neurological or biological basis there is little that can be done to control behavior except for medication or application of rigid approaches to manage the behavior. However, there is ample evidence that even biologically based behavioral problems can be greatly reduced and, in many cases, managed with enough success for a child to perform well at home and in school. For example, it has been shown that children with attention-deficit problems can be taught self-regulatory methods that significantly improve their ability to focus. In addition, many behavioral problems experienced by children can be improved by a simple change in the teacher or parent's attitude. Change may be brought about through increased understanding of the difficulties a child may have in managing frustration and stimulation and in regulating and organizing behavior.

Developmental factors

Developmental problems or delays, which may or may not have an identifiable neurological or biological basis, also can be a source of behavioral problems. Developmental disorders such as expressive language disorder often lead to social withdrawal, academic difficulties, and heightened frustration resulting in tantrums or outbursts. Other developmental disorders such as autism are diagnosed because of the existence of disruptive or unusual behaviors and social interactions. As with neurologically or biologically based behavioral problems, behaviors that reflect developmental delays or disorders can be significantly influenced by how the parent or teacher handles them; many conflicts can be effectively addressed with management techniques that reflect an understanding of the problem.

Children with behavioral difficulties should be properly screened for health problems. Vision and hearing deficits impede social and emotional development, speech and language development, and behavior; poor growth attributed to lack of nutrition may in fact be due to urinary tract infection or low thyroid levels. In either case, an early health screening can be critical to ensure each child has the opportunity to reach her full potential.

Emotional factors

A child's emotional problems can be a source of behavioral and learning problems. Many times the causes of difficulties such as anxiety, depression, anger, and hostility are not clear, though they often reflect other factors in the child's life, particularly problems deriving from the home environment. Children have difficulty handling stress in the home. They quickly become disorganized and do not understand their loss of control — they are confused and frightened by it. These children frequently are identified as "willfully disobedient" or "behavior problems" by the parent or teacher who may misunderstand the nature of the child's problem and increase the child's anxiety and stress. While disruptive behaviors often are the presenting picture of a child with emotional problems, it is important not to overlook other emotionally troubled children who present as withdrawn or quiet.

Motivational Factors

Many times children demonstrate behavioral problems because they are looking for a particular outcome. The parent or teacher that can identify the motivation behind a child's behavior (Table 9.1) will be able to adjust the environment or the relational interactions with the child and improve the child's behavior.

TABLE 9.1 MOTIVATIONAL FACTORS FOR BEHAVIOR	
Behavior	Motivation
Seeks control of events and situations	Power/control
Seeks to avoid a task, consequence, or negative situation	Protection/avoidance/escape
Tries to set self apart from others; wants to be the focus	Attention
Constantly seeks to relate to others	Acceptance/affiliation
Seeks forum for expression of needs, skills, or talents	Self-expression
Seeks self-directed reward or enjoyment	Gratification
Seeks settlement of differences; tries to "get even"	Justice/revenge

While behavioral problems may reflect motivational goals, it is important to remember that for some children behavior may emerge out of the child's effort to cope with a neurological or developmental vulnerability. When a child is behaving negatively, it is usually more productive for the parent or teacher to try to determine what the child hopes to achieve with the misbehavior than to engage in punitive measures. If a reason can be found, then interventions can successfully be developed to address the misbehavior.

Interactions between ecological and child-specific factors

Interactions between ecological factors and child-specific sources of disruptive behavior can create particular problems for the parent or teacher. When a child has a neurological predisposition to hyperactivity and inattentiveness (child-specific factor) and comes from a home in which the parents are not providing adequate structure and limit-setting for their child (ecological factor), the child may show the distractibility and impulsive behavior characteristic of a child with ADHD. For a child who resides in an unsafe neighborhood with few resources, these problems often are made worse. Certainly, there is a neurological basis for the child's behavior; however, it is likely the ecology of the home and neighborhood — including a lack of structure and routine, exposure to violence and danger, and inconsistent discipline — that is exacerbating his behavioral tendencies and making the problem worse.

Child abuse also reflects this interaction of ecological and child-specific factors. Often the child who is difficult to manage because of poor behavioral control is a target for abuse by a parent who has poor self-control. Overly punitive physical punishment, long periods of seclusion, or cruel, verbally abusive language can exacerbate a child's behavioral problems. It is not unusual for an abused child to exhibit a range of behavior problems that include both under-controlled and over-controlled patterns. In addition, patterns of oppositionality and defiance can emerge because the child does not trust adult authority. If the child moves from the biological home to a foster home, it is not unusual for the child to feel abandoned by the abusive family.

Children's misbehavior as a message

Traditional behavior modification approaches that stress reinforcement of good behavior and use time-out and cost response techniques to withhold reinforcement may be ineffective when used with certain children, especially those prenatally exposed to alcohol or illicit drugs, or those who have suffered early trauma. The children's self-regulatory difficulties, lack of ability to organize, and increased anxiety lead them to respond to the punitive nature of behavior modification interventions with heightened agitation. As a result, interventions such as time-out may backfire: the very behavior one wants to reduce is escalated as the child continues to discharge tension through inappropriate behavior. Far more effective for under-controlled children are preventive strategies that help children learn to self-regulate and provide positive incentives to encourage special effort on the part of the child.

Although it is common for adults to react to children's misbehavior by seeking to control, change, or eliminate it, it is more useful to consider misbehavior as a message that something is wrong (Table 9.2), which the child does not know how to correct. Usually the behavior is functional—that is, it helps the child cope with anxiety, anger, frustration, overstimulation, or other negative feelings. Accordingly, parents and teachers will be unsuccessful in eliminating it unless they help the child find alternative behaviors that are more appropriate or adaptive. However, this is not always easy, for children can send many messages through their behavior, and it may be difficult to determine what they are trying to communicate. For instance, a child who hits his teacher may be striking out, not out of anger, but frustration at his inability to understand an assignment. Usually, however, through experience with that child, the parent or teacher can read the message, figure out the behavior, and take some action. The important thing to remember is that a message is there, and if you can figure it out, you may well be on your way to solving the problem.

TABLE 9.2 BEHAVIORAL MESSAGES	
Behavior	Message
Withdrawal	"I'm scared." "No one likes me." "I'm sad." "I don't know how to reach out to others."
Shyness	"I'm overwhelmed." "I'm unsure of myself." "I can't cope with this."
Submissiveness	"I don't feel good about myself." "I don't know what to do."
Aggression	"I can't do this, it's too hard." "I'm not being treated fairly." "I'm frustrated." "I'm angry." "I can't cope with this."
Inattention	"I'm bored." "I don't know what to do." "I need a break." "I got distracted."
Refusal to comply	"I'm mad and I don't want to be here." "This is not fair." "If I try, I'll fail."
Non-completion of tasks	"I don't know how to do this." "This is too hard." "I don't know how to organize this." "I got distracted and forgot what I was doing."

The most important aspect of reading and responding to behavioral messages is the ability to empathize. This means successfully picking up on the message embedded in behaviors and responding with affirmation to that message and the function it serves. Empathic, reflective statements: "I see that you're angry about this," or "It seems like you're having trouble organizing this work by yourself," or "I know it was easy to be distracted by your sister's telephone call, but now let's see if we can focus on the work and remember what we need to do," can be very powerful interventions as they allow a child to feel understood and enhance her sense of trust and safety with that adult.

However, all of us can reach the point at which we feel unable to deal with the behavior problems that confront us. It is hard to feel empathy when we feel powerless, so we respond out of our own frustration. Empowerment—the degree to which we feel capable of dealing with the child's behavior, including the problems arising from negative or disruptive behavior—is critical. Parents and teachers who feel empowered are more likely than those who do not to engage in problem solving and respond in empathic, proactive ways. To that end, we must guard ourselves against feelings of frustration and anger that may cause us to react without reflection, thinking there is no solution to the problem and thereby complicating the child's existing difficulties. More often than not, there are solutions. Although we may be faced with complex, confusing, and heartbreaking behavioral and learning problems in our children, we must move beyond blaming the child to find solutions. That's what hope is all about.

PART III
THE LANGUAGE OF WHISPERS

The purpose of this section is to look at those quiet times when opportunities occur for behavioral management as well as therapeutic insight. All of the intervention strategies are based on the principles and information presented in the first two sections. There is no one simple recipe for improving a child's behavior. However, emerging evidence supports strategies that acknowledge the usefulness of behavior management techniques combined with mental health interventions. Just remember these key principles:

- Behavioral change occurs in the quiet moments. It does not happen as a consequence of yelling or fussing or cajoling or bribing, or in the heat of a crisis.
- Behavioral change is slow. It does not happen overnight, and it does not hinge on one specific moment. Behavioral change requires constancy, consistency, and support.
- Most of all, behavioral change must be anchored in the whispered connections between parent and child.

10 Coming to a Theatre Near You: The External Brain

Children's behavioral problems are related to a variety of factors. While you are not likely to find a cure-all intervention for behavioral problems associated with any one predisposing factor, many times a combination of strategies will be effective. The key is to look beyond the behaviors you see for the root cause of those behaviors. Whether or not a child was prenatally exposed to alcohol and drugs, the overall goal is to help children learn to manage themselves, rather than to rely on an outside source, such as the parent or teacher, to control their behavior. This chapter will present some fundamental principles of behavior management that are key to helping move children from external control to internal management.

Prosocial behavior

Prosocial behavior refers to the social and self-control skills a child needs to meet demands encountered in school, at home, and in the community. Developing prosocial behavior is an integral part of teaching a child behavior management and can have long-lasting effects. As an adoptive parent or teacher, you may encounter children who have not had an opportunity to learn social skills within their biological home environment. Families with substance use disorders often do not offer feedback on behavior, or the feedback does not include an alternative behavior that could be substituted appropriately for the unacceptable one. Rules and consequences are inconsistently administered, and children do not know what is socially appropriate because they have never had proper instruction. They lack the kinds of social problem-solving skills needed to guide them in making good choices as to how to behave.

Proactive approaches

When attempts to manage behavior are not complemented with equal effort to teach the desired behavior, there will be minimal benefit over the long term. In fact, if control of behavior only is achieved through punitive or negative approaches, it is very possible that behavioral problems will increase as the child retaliates. Punitive or negative approaches to behavior management actually make the behavior worse.

When children do not behave as expected, the reason may fall into one of two categories: skill deficits or performance deficits. The key to changing behavior may lie in addressing the reason a child does not comply with expectations.

Skill deficits

Skill deficits refer to the child's lack of skills to perform desired tasks. Reasons for skill deficits include faulty teaching and modeling of appropriate behaviors, reinforcement for inappropriate instead of appropriate behaviors, and the child's lack of opportunity to learn the desired skills. Some children may enter a classroom, or a foster or adoptive family, without ever having such simple experiences as hearing stories or rhymes, learning colors and numbers, or naming the objects in their environment. Vulnerable or high-risk children, in particular, may have more difficulty learning certain types of skills needed for prosocial behavior due to impulsive behavior, low frustration tolerance, and a tendency toward disorganized behavior.

TABLE 10.1 STEPS PARENTS AND TEACHERS CAN TAKE TO TEACH A CHILD PROSOCIAL BEHAVIOR
1. Provide opportunities for the child to have focused attention in the family or classroom conversation. Allow the child to be heard and to hear others sharing news from school, friends, and work in progress.
2. Be clear on rules and guidelines for expected ethical behaviors. Let the child participate in making rules about respectful interactions in the family or among her peers.
3. Model social situations and practice interpersonal problem-solving skills that can provide positive ways for the child to assert her needs, resolve conflicts, and make friends. Ask the child to consider goals and reflect on options and their consequences.   • "If someone calls you a name, what can you do?" "If you do that, what is likely to happen?"   • "If you need something and someone is using it for a long time and won't let you use it, what can you do?" "If you do that, what is likely to happen?"   • "If someone pushes you in line . . ."   • "If you want someone to play with and you are afraid to ask . . ."   • "If someone makes you very angry (or very happy) . . ."

For skill deficits, the challenge is to determine what the specific deficits are and to teach the child to counteract them. Typically, the child is not intentionally misbehaving; she simply is not equipped with the knowledge of what is appropriate. While for some children the skill deficits are small and need little remediation, other children will require substantial effort. For example, a young child at school who has difficulty lining up to go to lunch, or who cannot get her backpack together to get ready for school, may need to be physically walked through these processes until they become a part of her repertoire. Likewise, the girl who cannot complete work without someone working alongside her, or who gets sidetracked from her homework before bed, initially needs extra help organizing her work; then regular check-ins from the parent to ensure that she has kept herself on track. You will find that identification and remediation of skill deficits often will correct and eliminate problem behaviors. The child will know what to do and what is expected, especially when given well-placed reminders and positive reinforcement and praise.

TABLE 10.1 (*continued*) STEPS PARENTS AND TEACHERS CAN TAKE TO TEACH A CHILD PROSOCIAL BEHAVIOR
4. Model respect, friendliness, firmness of purpose, and interest through interactions with the child. • Show the child what you expect • Use affirming and encouraging language • Stress the deed, not the doer • Notice and comment on what the child does "right" • Redirect behavior using a firm, kind manner • Say what you mean, mean what you say
5. Provide opportunities to participate in group family activities and to learn to work together. • Divide and share tasks • Plan cooperative projects in the home • Organize group games for fun, not competition • Assign developmentally appropriate household chores
6. Provide opportunities for the child to learn constructive ways to handle controversy and differences. • Have family discussions of current events • Suggest different "right" solutions to the same problems • Hold family meetings to discuss and solve problems • Teach the value of diversity and acceptance

Performance deficits

Performance deficits refer to those skills that a child has and knows how to perform, but for a variety of reasons does not exhibit in practice. Often children have the skills to produce the desired behaviors, but interfering factors prevent them from being put into practice. To address performance deficits, one must understand why the child is not performing as desired, respond sympathetically to this problem, and convince the child that negative behaviors are inappropriate, and appropriate "prosocial" behaviors will lead to greater benefit.

Performance deficits are characterized by highly variable behavior in which a child does well in one setting but not in another. Certain locations may provide ecological dimensions that are missing elsewhere such as a level of structure, consistency, or personal interest that is well aligned with the child's needs. As you work with children, keep in mind that variability in performance also may indicate a skill deficit. The child may demonstrate skills when working with a therapist directly in a one-to-one situation, but when left to complete the same material on his own, he may be unable to do so because of organizational deficits. At times, the distinction between performance and skill deficits can be difficult to assess. However it is important to make this distinction because it will determine the correct intervention strategy.

The proactive approach to addressing a performance deficit is to identify an alternative, desired behavior and strengthen it through positive reinforcement, teaching the child to feel good about using the appropriate behavior. Although it may seem unnatural at first, the best approach is to de-emphasize or ignore the undesired behavior and focus on positive alternatives. Of course, ignoring behaviors can be difficult and at times impossible; in those situations, it is best to use techniques that minimize occurrences of bad behavior as you work to improve the child's self-control and social skills.

Management vs. control

Often when parents and teachers talk about managing a child, they equate it with maintaining control of the child. Control is taken to mean suppressing or containing undesirable behavior so instruction or family interactions can continue in an orderly manner. However, so much time is spent developing ways to externally control children's behavior that parents and teachers may fail to promote the children's taking control of their own behaviors. Children's self-control is achieved by facilitating their development and empowering them through respect, listening, collaboration, and problem-solving approaches. From this perspective, our goal is to maintain family or classroom activities while teaching children the tools to internally manage their own behavior.

> Cheryl was clearly frustrated as she related Warren's behaviors to our team's psychologist. "He gets into trouble

every day. He can't concentrate on what he's supposed to be doing. He seems to be going in five different directions at one time; then he starts running and in a few minutes he's running wild and screaming. Sometimes he pushes his brothers when they're in his way. I have no choice but to send him to his room and punish him. When I do that, though, he sulks for the rest of the day and won't come to dinner with the family. I tried taking away television privileges, but no matter how many times I do, he does the same thing again the next time he has the chance. None of his brothers want to play with him anymore because he has to control anything they play, which leads to fights and gets them all into trouble."

Cheryl's use of threats and confinement to interrupt Warren's behavior hasn't worked. The descriptions of Warren's behavior suggest he has trouble controlling his behavior and organizing himself. His mother has attempted to control him by sending him to his room. Although it may be necessary to remove him from a situation temporarily, he does not seem to be learning anything from it; the behavioral difficulties are repeated on an almost daily basis. This is the problem with strategies aimed at controlling rather than managing behavior—the child learns no self-control, no idea of how to act appropriately.

TABLE 10.2 REQUIREMENTS FOR CHILDREN TO MANAGE THEIR OWN BEHAVIOR	
Structure	A stable environment in which the child knows what is expected and how to go about doing it.
Predictability	A home and classroom in which the child knows what her day will look like and how her family and teacher will respond to her.
Consistency	An environment in which responses to the child are the same every day.

Another important lesson from Warren's case is that children may find it extremely difficult to manage blocks of free time.

The combination of excitement and lack of structure can make it challenging for the child to calm down and organize his behavior. Think *prevention*. Discuss expectations for play behavior prior to letting Warren go outside with his brothers. Set a clear plan for what he would like to do outside and with whom he would like to play, so there is structure for his activity. Talk through what his behavior should look like and what you will do if you notice his behavior is not in keeping with his stated plan. As soon as problems arise, Warren should be removed from the situation and provided an alternative location where he can calm down until he appears ready to manage his behavior again. Make sure to give Warren generous praise as he becomes increasingly successful in managing himself.

You will find that with time Warren may be able to take himself out of situations when he is beginning to feel out of control, giving himself a "break" in order to regain self-control. It is important to note that these strategies are in direct contrast to a "time-out," whereby a child is suddenly removed from a situation in the heat of a moment. Laying out the plan ahead of time and allowing the child to remove himself from the situation when he begins to feel out of control—what we call a "cool down"—is a proactive approach to teaching a child self-management.

> Trying to uncover some possible contributing factors for Warren's behavior, the psychologist asked about the previous evening. "Everything went OK after school until dinner time," Cheryl recalled. "My husband and I and the boys were eating and talking. Then Warren got up and started walking around the room, flicking his finger at everyone. I told him to sit down and eat his dinner, and he said he didn't like the food, even though I had asked him what he wanted for dinner. I told him that he would have to leave the room, so I sent him to his room and closed the door. He started making noises through the vent. I sent my husband to talk with him. When Warren

came back to the dinner table, he hit one of his brothers because he said he drank some of his milk. I'm afraid I lost my temper and told him that if he didn't want to eat I didn't care what he did as long as he didn't bother anyone else. Then he started making quacking noises, messing up everyone's dinner. I have told him that he'll have to eat alone from now on. I don't know what to do with him anymore. I have tried every punishment I know, and he doesn't seem to care!"

Here Cheryl is showing telltale signs of frustration. She appears to think Warren is acting out in order to bother her or the rest of the family. However, there are many possibilities to explain this behavior. Warren may be having difficulty focusing on the task of eating because of a distraction in the room or problems at school. The first indication that Warren was having trouble managing himself came when he left his seat and began to walk around the room. At that point, Cheryl could have checked to see that he understood that dinnertime was a time for the family to be together and share a meal. By inviting Warren back to the dinner table for another ten minutes, perhaps asking him to tell a story from his day at school, there is a good chance that escalation of the situation could have been avoided.

In this case, Cheryl makes the situation worse by assuming Warren is willfully misbehaving and using techniques to suppress and control behavior. Because Warren's distractibility and low tolerance for frustration seem to be at the heart of the problem, her efforts to control Warren by confrontation only rub salt in the wound. There are several alternative strategies that Cheryl could apply in the future to prevent the escalation of problems:

1. Listen carefully to Warren's communication and respond in a way that lets him know he has been "heard."
2. Recognize that not all challenging behavior is intentional acting out in pursuit of attention for attention's sake.

3. Adjust her communication style out of recognition that not all children operate at the same level, nor respond to formal explanations and directions in the same way.

4. Remember that there may be more than one explanation for a child's behavior—and seek out alternate possibilities.

5. Acknowledge the constant need for the parent to balance her responsibilities to the family as a whole and to the special needs of specific children.

TABLE 10.3 CONTRASTING CONTROL VS. MANAGEMENT OF BEHAVIOR		
Behavior	Control	Management
Warren gets into fights with his brothers.	Send Warren to his room.	Talk through the expected behavior with Warren before he plays with his brothers. Create a plan for behavior and activity, with a model for what he should do if he feels himself getting into trouble with the other children.
Warren leaves his seat and wanders around the room during dinner.	Keep Warren in his seat.	Make sure dinnertime is clearly organized and structured. Set a time limit for how long Warren is expected to be at the table (ten minutes, for example), then permit a short break before he returns for another ten minutes.
Warren needs to control the activity in games.	Keep Warren from fighting with his brothers.	Coach all children before play about sharing and control. Review expectations for behavior. Check on Warren regularly to provide extra coaching.
Warren withdraws when he feels he cannot succeed in a task.	Keep Warren from withdrawing.	Stress the goal of learning rather than success or failure in schoolwork. Never use humiliation when the child cannot perform. Teach siblings how to support each other's learning efforts.

Preventing behavior problems

Much of what is written and practiced in managing children's behavior targets emotional and behavioral problems that have a long history and may require direct interventions to modify. However, another important aspect of addressing problems is to learn more about preventing their occurrence in the first place. It is much more effective to prevent problems than to respond to them after they have emerged. In fact, many discipline strategies may escalate the difficulties children have in managing themselves:

- Chronic punishment or punishment without praise or positive feedback
- Absent, ambiguous, or inconsistently enforced behavior rules
- Inadvertent reinforcement of undesirable behavior
- Failure to recognize or reinforce desirable behavior when it occurs
- Practices that serve to embarrass, denigrate, humiliate, or intimidate a child such as threats; negative comments about the child's ability or characteristics (especially in the presence of peers); neglect for the child's needs; corporal punishment
- Lack of a comprehensive and effective plan for helping the child learn how to manage his behavior

In a nutshell, two key principles govern preventive behavior management: (1) promoting positive, desired behaviors and (2) minimizing disruptive behaviors. The home or classroom that is prevention focused will use procedures and techniques that focus on both components. Remember that even in the best-managed situations, where sound prevention practices are evident, problem behaviors nevertheless will occur.

Promoting and communicating desired behaviors
How often have you heard someone say, "You know better than that," to a child? Adults tend to assume that children have learned what is acceptable and what is unacceptable behavior when often

that is not the case. In working with children, we must not only tell them what we don't want them to do, but also be very specific in explaining why that behavior is unacceptable and what would be an acceptable alternative. Every time you talk to children about their behavior be sure to use clearly stated rules and expectations so they know what behaviors will earn a positive response. Although telling a child precisely what you want is the most logical way to communicate, you may try other ways to convey desired behaviors:

- Post a chart of family or classroom rules
- Give the child feedback about her behavior
- Show approval of her behavior through smiles, hugs, and other positive, nonverbal looks or gestures — catch her being good

Rules: A way to establish behavioral expectations

Communication of behavioral expectations provides clarity and consistency for what the child can expect and what she is expected to do. Children respect rules they have a hand in making, and generally learn more from rules that are positive and aimed at prevention. Rules should encourage reason and thinking and provoke active discussion. Though they may not always show it, young children want to please adults and be seen as "good" in their eyes.

Parents should be careful to apply the right measure of discipline when rules are broken. If a parent's response is too harsh, the child may experience a sense of shame that inhibits her initiative and capacity for autonomy. On the other hand, responses that are too weak may result in the child's not understanding how to control herself. For older children, eight to nine years old, rules are based on the well being of the social community. Issues of fairness, ethics, and the welfare of others are suitable for discussion. Most children at this age are capable of comprehending rules that apply beyond themselves to the needs of the group. They understand why such rules are reasonable and necessary.

Fair and consistent rules help establish a sense of order and control in the home or classroom and allow children to maintain a sense of control over their lives. Negatively stated rules, although easier to express than rules framed in the affirmative, imply an expectation of misbehavior. Parents are wise to avoid proscriptive rules that suggest what not to do, reserving them for innocuous occasions such as, "Don't bring toys to the dinner table."

Be consistent in what is expected and in how rules are enforced. If there is a rule

TABLE 10.4 RULES REGARDING BEHAVIORAL EXPECTATIONS
• Should be made and discussed with the children with a focus on why rules are needed.
• Should be made to serve a purpose.
• Should be stated in very clear, specific, and concrete behavioral terms. For example, rather than "Be nice to each other," a rule might be stated as, "Take turns with your brothers and sisters." Children should know when they are following a rule and when they are breaking a rule.
• Should be limited to no more than six (the fewer the better). They should be posted and easy to read.
• Should be stated in positive terms because this communicates positive expectations. Say what we do, not what we don't do.
• Should be discussed to see how they relate to daily routines and activities.
• Should be reviewed on a regular basis, e.g., every two weeks and whenever a member of the family or classroom violates a rule.
• Should be introduced prior to an activity to remind the children of expectations.

that a child should not interrupt his brother or sister, but it is not enforced when the child does interrupt, you can be certain it will be ineffective. One of the easiest ways to undermine the power of a rule is through inconsistency, so whenever a child violates a rule there should be a thorough discussion to ensure she understands it. Reminders or corrective statements for an individual child should be done in private, so as not to humiliate the child. Every so often it is a good idea to commend the child for her exceptional compliance with the rules by offering a special activity or reward.

Establishing a reward system

As a parent or teacher begins establishing a reward system, she must keep in mind that interruptions in expected rewards often cause uncertainty and confusion for younger children. If it becomes difficult to give rewards after positive behavior, then the procedures should be reviewed and revised.

TABLE 10.5 REWARDS FOR CHILDREN
• Should be logical and natural for the home or school environment
• Should be changed and varied, with higher behavioral requirements for rewards that are more highly valued (e.g., free time)
• Should be very specific and familiar, perceived to be attainable by the child
• Should be social as well as tangible (e.g., smiles, praise, privilege, recognition)
• Should be given consistently for positive behavior

First, identify rewards that the child can try to earn. Remember that what may be rewarding for an adult or older child may not be appreciated by the young child. Develop a list of rewards that students in a classroom or children at home prefer by asking them what incentives they appreciate, observing their behavior, and talking with other parents and teachers.

At first, reinforcement should be given each time a desired behavior occurs. Plan to gradually decrease the amount of reinforcement expected, and remind the child why she is receiving the reward. Even if a tangible reward is not given each time, social rewards such as praise can be given in their place. For younger children or children who regularly exhibit negative behaviors, the frequency at which you give rewards for appropriate behavior is particularly important.

Parents and teachers also must minimize rewards for inappropriate or undesired behavior. Although it may seem difficult to imagine anyone rewarding undesired behavior, this happens frequently. For example, an adult's conspicuous verbal reprimand may be perceived as a reward in the mind of the attention-hungry child who misbehaves in public. The parent's actions increase the likelihood the child will repeat the behavior because the child is rewarded for her misbehavior, earning the attention she was seeking.

So how do you prevent unintentional rewards? The easiest way is to observe the reaction of the child to the consequences you apply when undesired behaviors occur. Watch to see if the behavior increases and, if so, review your approach, considering how to respond to that child if the situation recurs. In general, it is a good idea to ignore mild occurrences of disruptive or negative behavior because acknowledging these will only fuel the fire, should the child perceive the attention as a reward. Of course, you will not be able to ignore extremely disruptive or dangerous behavior, and these issues should be addressed immediately and directly.

Using social reinforcers

Social reinforcers are events or actions between two or more people that serve to reinforce desired behaviors. They are convenient because they can be given quickly, require minimal effort, and can be used with groups or with individual children. Use of social reinforcers can have a dramatic effect by increasing desired behavior and reducing misbehavior. One important advantage of social reinforcers to other forms of behavioral modification is that children do not stop responding because they are tired of them. Properly used, social reinforcers can be a powerful tool in a parent's or teacher's repertoire of behavior management skills.

Although parents and teachers may not realize it, they use social reinforcers frequently, for instance whenever they say, "Great job," or "I like the way you're trying." To be effective, social reinforcers must be used in response to specific behaviors, rather than as a blanket statement about the child. Young children often do not know what it means to be a "good girl," but they appreciate recognition for a task done well. Social reinforcers may be even more useful if caregivers provide detailed and specific feedback to the child. Instead of saying, "Great job," try, "You did a great job paying attention and finishing your homework." Or instead of, "Good work," say, "I know it was hard for you to do that math homework, but you worked hard to get it finished."

Parents and teachers should be careful not to use verbal comments that appear reinforcing, but in reality are insulting. For example, saying something like, "You're a good student, but I'm disappointed in you because of this low math grade," may imply you are disappointed in the child as a person. A better way to respond to a child would be to say, "You've done well in math, but this assignment seemed to be giving you some trouble. Let's see what I can do to help you with these kinds of problems." This approach lets the child know you value her performance in math but recognize one area that gave her difficulty. There is no suggestion that the child is being criticized personally; instead, what is communicated is that this particular situation was troublesome, and you and the child can work together to improve performance. You are giving a social reinforcer, praise for having done well in math, but noting there is one area that needs attention.

Even in situations when some correction or help is needed, there are opportunities to give social reinforcement for positive behaviors exhibited by the child. When using social reinforcers remember that they should focus on behavior, they should be given immediately and often, and they should be clearly linked to observable behavior. Avoid the use of sarcasm at all times. No child should ever be embarrassed or humiliated.

Minimizing disruptive behaviors

> One afternoon I got a frantic call from Will's mother, Randi: "The teacher says if Will doesn't get put on Ritalin, she's kicking him out of class." Will had a long history of classroom difficulties, but the charm of his sandy hair and gap-toothed smile had kept him out of serious trouble. However, by third grade, his teacher was expecting more of him. "Can you tell me what happened?" I asked.

As she began again, Randi's voice was shaking: "From what I can understand, Will's teacher was in the middle of a lesson when Will jumped up and yelled, 'We have *Charlotte's Web* at home!' The class started laughing and acting up, and the teacher says he's out of her classroom unless he goes on Ritalin. I don't know what to do!" It appeared that Will's impulsiveness had gotten him into trouble again. "Let me call the teacher, if that's OK," I said. "Then we'll look at what's going on."

Children need a sense of control over their environment before they can feel confident in managing their own behaviors. That is why establishing daily routines can help prevent behavioral problems: a predictable schedule assists children in understanding and trusting their environment. Whether at school or at home, having clear expectations will reduce the anxiety children have in trying to organize their world.

I reached Will's teacher the next day. Over the phone I learned that the day before the incident, she'd taken the class to Chicago's Shedd Aquarium to see the dolphins. "We had a great time, and the next day everyone was still excited about the dolphins. So I started a session about dolphins. And it was one of those magical teaching moments when the whole class was with me, and I felt really good about the way things were going. Then all of a sudden Will jumps up and yells at the top of his voice, 'We have *Charlotte's Web* at home!'" As she said this, the energy drained from her voice. "The whole class started laughing and acting up. I lost them, and everything we had worked on that morning was lost. I'm tired of Will and his interruptions, and unless he gets put on Ritalin, he's not coming back to my class!"

We talked a bit more. Quite often, I request a behavioral log from a teacher, asking her to recall the exact circumstances and context of a specific behavior or incident. The log is as much a tool for recording the

child's behaviors, as it is a medium for teachers to record
their own actions and responses. In this case, the teacher
agreed to go back and track her interactions with Will that
day. A few days later a fax arrived with her behavioral
log.

Loss of behavioral control can be triggered by any number of
stimuli from a chaotic environment. In fact, anything that decreases
the predictability of the child's environment will increase the child's
self-regulatory problems. This is not just true for children with
prenatal substance exposure. Often children who display adequate
regulatory abilities in familiar environments lose this ability
when faced with a new set of circumstances, or during periods
of transition. However, with stable routines, rules, discipline,
and nurturing, children know what to expect from those around
them. Confidence in their environment gives children a sense of
stability, freeing them to focus on controlling their internal states of
arousal. The main point is that when children are exposed to new
environments or tasks, providing one-on-one attention, guidance,
and structure will help them maintain control.

Daily schedules

Daily schedules, whether at home or at school, provide consistency
to the child's life. Parents and teachers are wise to avoid changes
to the schedule. If the day needs to follow a different schedule,
each activity should be conducted but shortened. Variations from
routine such as vacations, schedule changes, and special events
produce anxiety and distrust in children and should be prepared
for appropriately. These simple strategies can help children control
and manage their behavior:

- Alternate quiet and active types of activities every twenty to
  thirty minutes, allowing for activities that will help the child
  burn energy.

- Post a daily and weekly calendar and review the day's schedule each morning.
- Provide closure at the end of the day. Discuss the next day and prepare for what will happen tomorrow.
- Be sure to advise the child ahead of time of any changes in the daily routine. Something as simple as a change in car pool arrangements can disrupt the child's ability to focus and stay on task for the rest of the day.

Transitions

Transitions often are unstructured and disorganized. Children who need a great deal of structure, or who have difficulty regulating their behavior in a chaotic or less-organized situation, will become lost as they move from one activity or setting to another. However, routines keep children occupied and involved; they are associated with enhanced achievement. Behavioral problems can be greatly decreased or prevented if simple strategies are applied:

- Introduce the structure of transition time to the children. Just like any other activity, transitions have a beginning, middle, and end.
- Provide clear cues or warnings to signal when a transition is about to begin, actually begins, and comes to end (e.g., music, timers, visual cues such as color codes and switching lights on and off). These cues are especially helpful at bedtime.
- Review the routine of a transition before it is to begin.
- Demonstrate and describe each step of a transition for children who require a great deal of structured guidance.
- Be sure to acknowledge any differences children may see or experience following the transition.

According to Melissa's behavioral log, the day had started out like any other. She had arrived early, gone to the teacher's lounge to collect her mail, and settled into her classroom to review her lessons and prepare for the day. However, on this particular day, a poster announcing publication of a new edition of *Charlotte's Web* had arrived in the mail. It was bright, attractive, and perfect for posting in a place of honor, next to the blackboard. She thumbtacked the poster up and awaited the arrival of her students.

Will sat in the classroom listening to the teacher, but was constantly pulled off task, wondering what the new poster was doing in the room. He tried to control himself, but the tension of trying to stay on task and shut out the distraction was too much. Eventually, the only way to relieve that tension was to jump out of his chair and acknowledge the presence of the poster. "We have *Charlotte's Web* at home!"

Could this have been prevented? Many teachers complain that they cannot make accommodations for any one child in a classroom. With the pressure of large class sizes, the demands of standardized testing, and the high level of responsibility placed upon them by the community, teachers argue that addressing the needs of one child in the classroom is too time consuming. While it may appear to be a good idea in theory, it is quixotic, impractical, and unfair to other students—a wasted effort in the larger scheme of things. But, in fact, Will's case is a telling example of how little things can help maintain order in a classroom, not just for one student but collectively. The poster was brand new. Most likely, several children were wondering about it and being pulled off task.

We can assume the better-regulated children in the class were able to habituate to the presence of the poster and focus on the lesson at hand. However, Will, because of his regulatory difficulties, could not put that poster aside. He had no way to release the mounting tension he was feeling until he jumped out of his chair. The teacher could simply have said, "Class, today we're going to talk about dolphins. But I want to show you a new poster on *Charlotte's Web*, a book that we're going to read soon. But today, it's all about dolphins." In this way, she would have put the poster into the context of the classroom, helping all the children in the class focus and attend to the day's lesson. Most important, it would have relieved the tension that Will was feeling and kept him in his seat.

In telling Will's story, my point is neither to single out Melissa, nor to carp on teachers for what is no doubt an immensely challenging job. Instead, I borrow Will's story to show the tendency in some homes or classrooms to try to fit the child to the typical routine, rather than the other way around. Routines are important but this does not mean that traditional practices set up for the family or classroom should become so inflexible they cannot be modified to meet a particular child's needs. Fitting a round peg in a square hole simply will not work, and sometimes parents and teachers need to take a step back and examine the situation with prudence. Common sense presumes some level of modification in policy and practice in the best interest of the child.

The pain of homework

The home is the environment in which the parent interacts with the child and where the child spends most of her time. Unfortunately, as the child gets older, demands of homework can bring the pressures of school into the home and precipitate confrontations between the parent and child. To make homework a much less difficult time for everyone in the family, there are several steps you may take as a parent:

- Give your child a "learning corner" at home to go to when she needs to work on school assignments. Doing homework at the kitchen table, in the midst of household activities, is a set-up for problems. Be sure the child's work area is free of distractions, including radios and televisions. Use a fan or some other source of "white noise" to block out other sounds around the house. Have a favorite chair or blanket near the child's desk or work space so that when she starts to feel overwhelmed she can get away from the cause of her anxiety.

- Keep to a set schedule as much as possible. Start homework at the same time each day. Establish routines in coming home from school, enjoying some "down time," getting ready for working on the school assignments, having dinner, and completing homework. Prepare your child well in advance for any changes from that routine.

- Pay special attention to transition times. Children with problems organizing their behavior often will have difficulty moving from one activity to another. Give your child a warning at least ten minutes ahead of time when it is time to stop working and come to dinner.

- Avoid the rush of last minute pressures. Include long-term homework assignments on a weekly calendar. Teach your child to plan and track progress toward completion of assignments, and let her check them off when completed.

Essentially, by following these strategies, you become your child's "external brain." You are teaching the child strategies for organizing, planning, and completing a task, the higher order executive functioning skills discussed in chapter 5 that utilize all aspects of the brain and which research has shown are crucial to a child's long-term development. Children who have good executive functioning skills in the first grade will continue to do well over the course of the life span, while children who have difficulties with executive functioning have difficulty in school and are at high risk for significant social and learning problems as they get older. The key is routine. By providing consistent guidance and prompting in a loving, non-confrontational manner, you can help your child to improve her capacity for executive functioning.

Utilizing contingencies and logical consequences

Although reward systems may help to promote positive behavior, parents and teachers often must adopt more active approaches to minimize undesired behaviors. One approach that is successful in children as they reach school age is the use of contingencies and logical consequences.

Contingencies are central to effective behavior management. The best synonym for "contingency" is "dependent" and refers to the relationship of one event to another. If there is a contingent relationship between two events, then one results from the occurrence of the other. For example, an adult receives a paycheck contingent (dependent) upon her working, a student receives an "A" grade contingent upon doing the necessary work at a high quality, and a child receives a reward contingent upon whether she completes a task for which the reward has been promised.

Many parents and teachers are uncomfortable with the idea of using rewards to help children manage their behavior, believing that rewards are a form of bribery. But when used with discretion incentives can be a powerful intervention that sends the message: "You [the child] are in charge of what happens, I am not controlling you—it's up to you." Thus the parent or teacher, rather than being seen as the evil sovereign of punishment, becomes the coach who can empower the child to exert control and manage himself.

Incentives also are a way to acknowledge that you are asking a child to do something that is difficult for her. In many ways, incentives for children are no different from the kinds of incentives and bonuses provided to adults in the workplace when employers want more productivity. When you offer an incentive for successful execution of a task understood to require great effort, you provide an empathic show of support that lets a child know you understand him and do not blame him.

Positive incentives are an especially useful tool with children who are oppositional or defiant, because they give the child an opportunity to choose good behavior that will be rewarded. They are also ideal for children who tend to be impulsive. For these children, the wish to act occurs almost simultaneously with action itself and making a different choice requires additional mental processing. Incentives help a child put a couple of beats between the wish to act and the action (e.g., "If I hit this kid, I'll lose my sticker"), and strengthen the child's capacity for self-control.

Using these types of interventions also allows the parent or teacher to be creative in his involvement with the child. What motivates the child? How can the contingency be structured? How can the child work to meet extra goals? Remember, the chosen contingency must be meaningful to the child—it must be something she wants in order to provide the motivation and incentive needed to reach the goal.

Parents reluctant to reward children may be pleased to learn that the world contains countless examples of contingencies that influence or manage behavior. Every day we receive rewards as a function of our behavior, for example, the "thank you" we get for offering a houseguest a glass of water. And who hasn't received negative consequences for inappropriate behavior, say, a traffic ticket for speeding? Obviously, then, not all contingencies are positive. Often a child will earn attention from a subset of his peers for acting aggressively—the attention contingent upon his being aggressive. In reality, a contingency by itself is neither positive nor negative: it is the nature of the relationship that is important.

Contingencies also can be viewed as logical consequences that teach children to take responsibility for their own behavior. Logical consequences are effective because they link a behavior with its repercussions, reinforcing the habit of self-regulation in the child's mind.

TABLE 10.6 GUIDELINES TO ENHANCE THE SUCCESS OF LOGICAL CONSEQUENCES
• Logical consequences make sense and are connected to the misbehavior.
• Logical consequences are respectful of the child. The child is allowed a voice in the discussion of possible consequences, including a stake in determining the details of the consequences.
• Logical consequences are not intended to humiliate or hurt.
• Logical consequences respond to choices and actions, not character. The message is that misbehavior results from poor judgment or bad planning but not from a fl aw in character.
• Logical consequences are put into practice with both empathy and structure. Empathy shows our knowledge of children and our willingness to hear what they have to say; structure establishes appropriate directions. The parent or teacher needs to be firm and kind. Kindness shows respect for the child; firmness shows respect for oneself.
• Logical consequences describe the demands of the situation, not the demands of the authority figure. This helps avoid power struggles.
• Logical consequences are used only after the parent or teacher has assessed the situation thoroughly. Misbehavior may result from expectations that are not appropriate to the developmental needs of the child, or from expectations incompatible with the child's particular needs. The best alternative may be to restructure the environment and readjust the expectations. When confronted with misbehavior, there are two questions to ask: a. Are my expectations appropriate to the age of the child? b. Are my expectations appropriate to the individual needs and abilities of the child?
• Logical consequences are imposed only after taking time to stop and think. It is important not to react suddenly.
• Logical consequences help to restore self-respect because self-respect demands not just words, but action.

Case Study: **Ronnie**

Ronnie is a third-grader who has difficulty completing all his homework due to visual-motor problems and attention deficits that make it hard for him to copy the ten sentences assigned each night by the teacher. His homework problems result in power struggles at home, with Ronnie usually going to bed feeling defeated and angry and his parents frustrated and at a loss for how to help. Despite suggestions by an outside psychologist, Ronnie's teacher refuses to modify the number of sentences Ronnie has to copy in order to receive credit for completion. At school, Ronnie displays disruptive behavior that is becoming more and more difficult for the teacher to manage.

1. What logical consequences is the teacher using?
2. Why is this likely to backfire?

Case Discussion

This teacher had a clearly defined policy that no child could be exempted from the expected work in her classroom. But what did the teacher and Ronnie gain from this rule—what logical consequence is she applying? Ronnie's failure to complete the assignment jeopardized his sense of competence, provoked his increasing anger and frustration, and led to behavioral problems requiring the teacher's attention and energy. If, instead, the teacher had considered the situation logically, modifying Ronnie's assignment to match his capabilities, Ronnie would have had a better opportunity for success. As for the teacher, she would have been able to give him positive feedback and not have had to engage in intrusive behavior management techniques. The wish to apply rules equally to all students is misplaced when the logical consequences of these rules impair the success of the children and the classroom.

While teachers may believe that adapting assignments for individual children will mean more work for them, preventive efforts like these almost always save time and energy later on. If Ronnie's teacher were to make accommodations for Ronnie and reduce the amount of work he was required to complete at home, there is a good chance his academic confidence would increase, limiting his classroom disruptions.

This case also points out the importance of the partnership between home and school. One of the best predictors of academic success for children is the degree to which parents are involved in the child's schooling. Although most parents value education and are aware that it is essential for their child's success, many feel unqualified to act in partnership with the school or to help their children academically because of negative experiences they had had when in school themselves. On the opposite side are teachers who too often blame parents for children's misbehavior, assuming that behavior is learned and that a child's misbehavior is obviously the fault of poor, inadequate, or indifferent parenting.

Even though it may be difficult at times, the single most important thing parents and teachers can do is to maintain an open line of communication:

- Parents should call the child's new teacher during the first month of school to introduce themselves, or send a letter or e-mail letting the teacher know when and where she may reach them if there is a problem.
- Parents should participate in routine conferences.
- Parents and teachers should compose two-way, home/ school communication notes about the child's progress.
- Parents need to let the teacher know when the child may be upset about circumstances at home. Teachers need to seek information about the child's progress, and should not necessarily compare this information against the rest of the class.
- Parents and teachers should communicate with one another about any problems a child has completing class work or homework, and work together in addressing these problems.
- Parents and teachers should communicate around celebratory events such as class parties, as well as for difficult situations such as disciplinary matters.

Behavioral concepts to guide management interventions

Two traditional tools widely used by parents and teachers to manage behavior are reinforcement and punishment. Reinforcement and punishment can be thought of as two ends of the same stick. Reinforcement seeks to affect behavior and learning by increasing a desired behavior or response so that it is more likely to occur. On the other side is punishment, which seeks to decrease the occurrence of an inappropriate or undesirable behavior.

Reinforcement

Reinforcement takes place when something the child likes, such as a novelty sticker or verbal praise, increases the frequency of an appropriate behavior. When the desired behavior occurs, the reinforcer (sticker, praise) must follow it. If the behavior increases in frequency or duration after the reinforcer is given, then reinforcement has occurred. Reinforcers include everything from material items to privileges, attention, praise, power, and choices.

Punishment

Punishment is used to decrease the occurrence of an inappropriate or undesirable behavior. When a child is making noises at the dinner table, the parent may reprimand her in an attempt to stop or decrease the behavior. If the child stops making noises after the reprimand, or makes the noise less frequently, then the reprimand is an effective punishment. Time-outs, verbal reprimands, and extra homework are all examples of punishment.

Punishment often does not provide an effective intervention because it increases tension and anxiety in the child and causes an escalation of the undesired behavior. Although time-outs can be an effective intervention for reducing unwanted behavior, for many children they elevate the arousal level, making it more difficult for a child to relax and reorganize his behavior.

Positive and negative reinforcement and punishment

There are two broad classes of interventions utilizing the reinforcement/punishment model: (1) positive reinforcement/ positive punishment and (2) negative reinforcement/negative punishment. Within this framework, positive means the act of providing something in response to a behavior, either a reinforcer (sticker) or punishment (extra homework), while negative means removing something.

Positive reinforcement

Positive reinforcement occurs when an event or object the child likes is given following an appropriate behavior, thus increasing the frequency of the behavior. Here positive reinforcement occurs because the frequency of the appropriate behavior increases in response to the presence of the reinforcer.

> Jamal and his mother are at odds. Jamal complains that his mother is always picking on him. His mother complains that Jamal is constantly running around and disturbing his brother and sister, instead of doing his homework. Because Jamal is interested in his baseball card collection, his mother works out a system in which Jamal earns points for every homework assignment he turns in on time. His mother exchanges the points for money that Jamal can use to purchase baseball cards. Jamal completes his homework on time.

Positive punishment

Positive punishment occurs when a disliked event or object is introduced to the child to reduce the occurrence of an inappropriate behavior. Here positive punishment occurs because the coach seeks to decrease the frequency of the behavior through the presence of punishment.

Eric is playing around and not listening to the coach
during practice. The coach tells him to do fifty push-ups
because of his inappropriate behavior.

Negative reinforcement

Negative reinforcement occurs when an event or object the child
dislikes is removed after the child demonstrates the appropriate
behavior. In this example, negative reinforcement occurs because
the frequency of the appropriate behavior increases in response to
the removal of the unwanted prompt.

Tom fails to complete class assignments independently
that his teacher knows he is capable of doing on his
own. The teacher stands near his desk, prompting him
to complete the work. Tom does not like the teacher's
frequent prompts, but he begins completing his work. In
turn, the teacher leaves him alone, and he continues to
finish his work to avoid future prompting.

Negative punishment

Negative punishment occurs when a desired event or object is
removed, resulting in a decrease in unwanted behavior. Removing
privileges, the most common use of negative punishment, can be
effective in the short term for reducing misbehavior. Here negative
punishment occurs because the teacher attempts to decrease an
undesirable behavior by removing a desired event or response.

Tamara continually talks to her friends during class,
despite frequent reminders to stop. The teacher punishes
her by not allowing her to go outside during recess.

CASE STUDY: **Sylvia**

Sylvia is constantly interrupting and parroting you. How would you handle this situation? Is your first impulse to punish Sylvia by taking away something she values, or would you seek to reward her for waiting to speak or speaking appropriately? Do you tend to use reinforcers or punishment? Positive or negative?

Case Discussion

While each form of intervention is effective in the short term, engaging Sylvia in a social problem-solving activity that asks her to think about why interrupting and parroting you cannot be tolerated would make the strongest impression in the long run. Ask her to brainstorm how you can help her better manage her impulsive behavior. Provide Sylvia with some initial suggestions or possibilities, including positive reinforcement (e.g., class participation points) for not talking out or negative punishment (e.g., loss of her recess privilege) if she interrupts more than a certain number of times in a given time period.

CASE STUDY: **Keisha**

Keisha is noisy and disruptive in the hallway on her way to computer class. How would you react in this situation? Assuming Keisha enjoys computer class, would you use negative punishment to keep her out of class? Or would you establish a contract with Keisha, awarding her points toward a desired activity (i.e., positive reinforcement) when she successfully negotiates transitions?

Case Discussion

Keisha may become hyper and over-stimulated during transitions and have difficulty managing her behavior. You might be able to improve her skills in this area by discussing the upcoming transition beforehand, then walking with her and holding her hand until she is calm enough to control herself effectively.

Integrating behavior management strategies

In the language of behavior management, any event following a behavior is a consequence, whether it is reinforcement or punishment. However, the effects of punishment, especially positive punishment, are unpredictable and often counterproductive when working with many children. On the other hand, logical consequences usually have a positive effect on children, not because these consequences punish or reward, but because they help children look more closely at their behavior. To put it another way, while rules help guide children to interact with their environment in a safe and orderly fashion, logical consequences allow children to internalize strategies of self-control.

A final concept to keep in mind as reinforcement and punishment are considered is the contingency, or connection, between a stimulus (e.g., a positive reinforcement) and the appropriate behavior. Receiving positive reinforcement is contingent on the child's performing the appropriate behavior. Understanding this contingency relationship and the difference between a contingency and a consequence will be important when you develop interventions. Children should never be given consequences unless they have been told ahead of time what to expect and can make the choice to control their behavior appropriately. When the child is put in the position of understanding the dependent relationship between the reinforcement or punishment and its behavioral antecedent, then the consequence becomes a contingency.

CASE STUDY: Jake

Jake is teasing his sister. His father tells him to stop but Jake continues to tease her. His father again says, "Stop teasing your sister." Jake ignores his father's request. Finally, Jake's father says, "I've had enough; out of here!" He sends Jake to his room for punishment.

Case Discussion

Although this reaction to Jake's teasing is a consequence of Jake's behavior, it is not a contingency. Had his father said the first time, "Jake, if you continue to tease your sister you will be asked to leave the room," he would have set up the contingency and given Jake a chance to make a choice and take responsibility for his own behavior. However, by applying a consequence without explaining its rationale, the power of the contingency is lost: the father has not allowed Jake to make the choice of what he will do. Establishing contingencies is especially important for children because it empowers them to make choices about, and thus learn to regulate, their own behavior.

These basic concepts—reinforcement and punishment, logical consequences, and contingencies—form the nucleus and grounding philosophy for behavioral intervention with children. They are especially important for substance-exposed children who have short-term memory deficits and difficulties connecting causes to their effects, because they form an immediate and logical consequence to behavior. Parents and teachers must look beneath the surface of the child's behaviors to try to understand the source of those behaviors. This will make application of behavior management strategies much more tenable for the child and much more successful for the adult.

11   Problem Solving as Opposed to Tearing Your Hair Out

A child's misbehavior can create chaos for a family or a classroom, and parents and teachers often fear that by devoting time and energy to a child with behavioral problems they will neglect their other children. The guilt, disappointment, and frustration that come with every new incident can cloud the best intentions of even the most caring mothers, fathers, and teachers, who often find themselves reacting to a situation rather than thinking it through. In these circumstances, a structured and systematic approach to behavior management is needed. The key concepts of reinforcement and punishment, logical consequences, and contingencies form the basis for a structured, problem-solving approach for behavior management.

The problem-solving approach ensures an objective, systematic method for determining which interventions are most appropriate for a given circumstance. It understands behavioral management issues as

TABLE 11.1 THE PROBLEM-SOLVING APPROACH	
Step 1	Identify target behavior
Step 2	Collect baseline data
Step 3	Establish contributing factors
Step 4	Identify appropriate bahavior to replace the target behavior
Step 5	Brainstorm possible interventions
Step 6	Communicate interventions to the child
Step 7	Implement selected interventions
Step 8	Evaluate and revise interventions

challenges to be solved sequentially in a series of steps. As shown in Table 11.1, practice involves monitoring the child's behavior, adapting interventions to the individual style and needs of both the parent and the child, evaluating the success or failure of your efforts, and revising them accordingly.

STEP 1: **Identify target behavior**

Children are not simple, and they usually present a range of behaviors that challenge parents and teachers. Typically, complaints come from parents who insist the child is "difficult about everything." Problems often include a combination of academic failure, inability to complete work, difficulty working independently and in groups, oppositional behavior, and bad temper. Parents describe their children as "difficult," "challenging," or "impossible," without providing a specific account of observed behavior. Thus, the first step in addressing difficult behaviors is to identify, specifically and in observable ways, the behavior that needs to be changed. Understand, we cannot suggest interventions that will make a child less "difficult," but we can talk about how to help a child be more compliant, better able to complete his homework, and less inclined to hit others when frustrated or angry.

Disruptions often are isolated in nature and can be dealt with on the spot. Sometimes the situation is very clear, such as when a child calls his sister a name. This can be handled with a simple, "Take it easy, Juan." However, when this type of behavior is repeated, you should identify it as a target behavior.

Identification of a target behavior can be guided by a series of questions:

1. Can you specifically name the behavior and document how often it occurs and how long it continues?
2. Could you describe the behavior to teachers or other parents so they know exactly what you mean (e.g., "Does not finish dinner")? If someone asks you what you mean, it

may indicate you are not yet specific enough. Even in this example, you might need to add more information (e.g., "Does not finish dinner in the allotted time").

3. Does the child understand what you are asking him to do?
4. If a teacher or another parent were to observe the child or behavior in question, would she agree with you about the behavior and its severity?

The more specific you can be in answering these questions the more effective you will be in managing the child's difficult behaviors. You will find yourself getting "stuck," if you have not defined the problematic behaviors with detail and precision. If this happens, return to this first step to clarify the difficulties the child is presenting. If you have trouble specifying those behaviors, try sitting down with your spouse or teachers who work with the child and have them ask you questions about the problems until they begin to take a more concrete form.

CASE STUDY: Tawanda

Tawanda's behavior is generally annoying. She talks continually and constantly interrupts you and her siblings. What behavior do you want to target?

Case Discussion

You can't target "annoying" without specifying it more clearly. The target behavior has to be specific and observable, and it must occur repeatedly. Based on the information above, you should target Tawanda's frequent talking and constant interruptions.

CASE STUDY: Chris

You find yourself disciplining Chris much more in public settings than at home. You know Chris gets into mischief during transition times and free time more often than during structured family activities. Since "mischief" is not a measurable behavior how might you identify behaviors that reflect Chris's disciplinary problems?

Case Discussion

Start by noting exactly what Chris is doing that is problematic. Each time you discipline him make a mental note of his behavior, including where and when it occurs. Over time you find these consistently occurring behaviors:

- "Jostling" others when he is in a crowded public place
- Not responding when he's asked to get ready to change activities
- Ignoring requests to "lower his voice" and "quiet down"
- Running around and having trouble settling down when arriving at a new location, such as the grocery store

The target behavior should be Chris's getting excited and out of control, especially during transitions.

STEP 2: Collect baseline data

Once you have identified specified behaviors you want to change, it is time to collect baseline data. The term "baseline" refers to the level of a behavior before intervention. Taking a baseline allows you to examine the severity of the child's problematic behaviors, from the onset, ensuring an objective picture of the intervention's effectiveness. Adults have a wide range of attitudes and responses to situations; we can be affected by the way a child looks, the child's family background, how well the child is liked, and the child's personality and attitudes. Baseline data answer the question, "Do I really see what I think I see?"

Baseline data also allow you to contextualize your observations. Often intervention should be immediate, and will not require a long-term problem-solving process. Other times behaviors may occur sporadically or inconsistently, making it difficult to determine their severity. However, if a behavior occurs with enough frequency to warrant a more elaborate intervention, you will need to establish the context in which the behavior occurs. Collecting baseline data, therefore, is not only about the child's behavior but also about what is happening in the child's surrounding environment, whether this is the classroom, home, or grocery store. The context in which the behavior occurs is critical.

Another way baseline data may be useful is as a tool for demonstrating to a skeptical teacher, parent, or spouse that a problem exists. Nearly every parent has had the experience of talking about a child's behavioral problem with a spouse who fails to recognize or believe there is a problem. The same can be said for teachers in their discussions with parents. Obtaining adequate baseline data mediates these disputes by providing documentation and justification for intervention.

Most important, collecting a baseline shows you whether an intervention is having any benefit by serving as a measuring device to evaluate changes in behavior. Give the intervention two to three weeks, then re-collect data on the targeted behaviors. If you collected good baseline data, then you will be able to compare your before and after numbers and determine whether your intervention has modified the targeted behaviors and, if so, by how much. That is valuable information to guide future interventions as new problems develop.

How might you go about collecting baseline data on behavior? First, remember the specific behaviors you have targeted and record them in a chart, with room for your dated observations. Begin to observe the child carefully to get a sense of the behaviors you wish to target, establish objective criteria for identifying the behaviors, and record them in terms of frequency, duration, severity, and context.

Frequency of behavior
You can establish baseline frequency simply by keeping track of how often the targeted inappropriate behavior occurs within a specific time period. For example, how often is a child off task during one

hour of independent work at his desk? How often does a child jump up from the dinner table? Frequency may be measured by counting all the occurrences of the behavior during a selected time period, such as an hour, day, or week, or by taking a sample during several different time periods. For example, instead of counting the number of times the child hits someone during a three hour period, you could observe the child's behavior for two or three minutes at a time. This method of sampling, if done well, will give a good approximation of the frequency of behavior without diverting too much of your time from other matters.

When evaluating frequency of behavior, be sure the behavior is not being caused by something unusual in the child's environment, such as the unexpected arrival of a guest, or a visit from a sibling's friend. You can use any convenient system to gather frequency data. Consider keeping a tally on a sheet of paper that describes the targeted behaviors, using note cards or a Microsoft Excel spreadsheet, or improvising with a method of your own.

Duration of behavior

Another way to establish baseline information is to assess how long a behavior lasts. Rather than counting the number of times a child is off task while doing homework, determine how long the child is off task within a given period. If the child was off task for three minutes out of five, then the duration of the inappropriate behavior would be 60% for that period. You can take several samples to verify that off-task behavior is occurring during other time periods and under a variety of circumstances. Duration recording is useful for behaviors that occur continuously rather than behaviors that are intermittent, such as staring out the window or not working independently.

Severity of behavior

Several standardized severity rating scales can be used to assess a child's behavior. Generally, results represent the parent's composite impression of a child's behavior over time. You can consult with your school's psychologist to determine what scales might be useful to you, or devise your own approach with simple criteria such as mild, moderate, and severe.

Because behavior and the perception of its severity are affected by an individual's subjective experience, the need to be objective when collecting these kinds of data is critical. What is considered disruptive or inappropriate in one environment may be viewed very differently in another. Each parent or teacher brings to his child rearing or teaching style his own tolerance level, expectations, and preferences. There may be times when a child is labeled as "uncontrollable," though clearly this is not true. It is easy for perceptions to be confused with reality and for children to be blamed for problems that may reflect skill deficits rather than defiance.

Context of behavior

In addition to using the strategies discussed above to establish a baseline, you also need to establish when the behaviors occur in order to put them into context. Think about the behaviors you've noted: Do the difficult behaviors occur first thing in the morning, after school, at the end of the day, or right before lunch? What tends to trigger the targeted behavior? Is it an interruption in the daily routine, another child in the family getting into trouble, the mother working with another child? Can you begin to predict when you will be most likely to observe the targeted behavior and, if so, what is the context in which it occurs? By understanding a behavior within an environmental context, you may find that the home or classroom is actually contributing to the problem. Perhaps you notice that each time Tory is off task while doing his homework he is looking at the constantly moving model airplane hanging nearby. Tory may in fact be off task because of a distraction in the room; removal of that distraction may resolve the attention difficulties he is displaying.

CASE STUDY: **Tawanda**

You decide to target Tawanda's talking and interruptions to determine if these behaviors are the source of your irritation with her. How would you determine if your belief is actually supported by fact? How can you be sure your own bias does not influence your general feeling of annoyance toward this child?

Case Discussion

Pure numerical data likely will support or invalidate your perception. Counting the frequency of Tawanda's interruptions (e.g., how many interruptions occur in various one-hour periods) will provide an objective view of how often she interrupts conversations. To develop a baseline for her talking behavior, record the percentage of minutes she talks during various periods in the school day. Make sure to include observations that describe the circumstances and time of day Tawanda's talking occurs.

CASE STUDY: **Chris**

You decide that Chris's target behaviors include those that indicate he is overly excited and having trouble calming down, especially during transitions. How do you document his behavior in a systematic fashion?

Case Discussion

Set up a behavior log to determine what kinds of behaviors are exhibited and at what times — baseline data. Record Chris's behavior each time you have to discipline him, noting what activity is occurring at this moment, and describe exactly what Chris is doing to draw your attention. You may also want to note what you did in response to his behavior and whether it had a positive impact. You should collect the data for at least a week.

STEP 3: **Establish contributing factors**

The problem-solving approach requires you to consider the multiple biological and environmental factors that contribute to the inappropriate behaviors you are seeing in the child. Contributing factors are either *proximal* — and have a direct and close relationship to current problems — or *distal*, contributing to current problems indirectly.

Proximal factors include developmental status, learning disabilities, skill deficits, medical problems, emotional or psychological problems, poor frustration tolerance, low tolerance for stimulation, the environmental qualities of the home, family events, and medications for medical or psychiatric problems.

Distal factors cannot be changed because usually they are associated with the child's environment and past history. The socioeconomic status of the family, the parents' use of illegal drugs, and prior abuse to the child all fall in this category. While often little or nothing can be done about these factors, they are an important part of understanding the function and meaning of the child's behavior, and at times you may be able to improve behavior by modifying their effects. For example, suppose a child with emotional problems tends to withdraw when a teacher criticizes his work. Often this is due to a history of being severely criticized at home: the child has learned to withdraw as a way to cope with criticism. The distal contributing factor is the child's past treatment, which the teacher cannot change. However the proximal contributing factor is how the child reacts to criticism. The teacher can assume a more relaxed tone, eliminating any use of strident or cutting remarks, to reduce the child's tendency to withdraw and increase his participation in classroom activities.

The first step in evaluating contributing factors is to gather information from observations of the child. Since you've collected baseline data, you probably already have some idea about when the problem behavior occurs. This knowledge will allow you to hypothesize what is going on, but fully understanding the factors that contribute to a child's behavior will require an open talk with the child. Throughout the conversation consider immediate factors in the child's life, such as a recent move into a new foster home, family illness, death, marital problems, or changes in household composition that put the child's behavior in context and allow you to choose an informed solution. Evaluate these factors in a nonjudgmental, respectful manner and talk with the child calmly, listening carefully to what he has to say. Through this conversation you may learn of distal factors bothering the child that were not immediately apparent.

CASE STUDY: **Tawanda**

You have collected baseline data on the frequency of Tawanda's interruptions at home and talked with her teacher to document the amount of time she spends talking at various points in the school day. You have recorded a range of observations about the situations in which these behaviors occur. What contributing factors might be influencing Tawanda's behavior?

Case Discussion

Evaluating the baseline data, you learn that Tawanda's most frequent interruptions at home occur when you are talking on the telephone or putting Tawanda's younger brother to bed. You talk to Tawanda's teacher and learn that Tawanda talks more often at school during math class than other subject areas, disturbing the work of other students by peeking at their papers or asking them questions. Interruptions and Tawanda's leaving her seat occur most frequently when the teacher is working with another student, or when she calls on another student during a class discussion. Tawanda's talking increases during field trips, assembly programs, and similar events that involve a high level of activity and excitement.

CASE STUDY: **Chris**

Baseline data verify your perception that Chris has trouble managing himself whenever structure in the home is reduced, especially during transitions from one activity to another or when given free time to play. Under these conditions, Chris becomes overly excited, exhibits poor self-control, and has trouble calming down. What are the contributing factors that may affect Chris's transition problems?

Case Discussion

You go to school and talk with Chris's kindergarten teacher, who, confirming Chris's difficulty with transitions, says he does not like changes of any sort and gets "wild." You know that as a younger child, changes in routine, particularly those involving highly stimulating situations, were very difficult for Chris to manage. Chris's baseline information indicates he is slow to change from one activity to another: about 50% of the time he is not ready for the new activity. Chris also appears to have difficulty when his "space" is invaded, whether in the back seat of the car, in line at school, or in the elevator during a field trip. In these situations, he becomes overexcited and aggressive and 70% of the time ignores requests to quiet down.

STEP 4: **Identify appropriate behavior to replace the target behavior**

Since most behaviors serve a function for the child, it is very difficult to eliminate or change them without providing a substitute that can serve the same function. That does not mean you cannot have clear rules about the unacceptability of certain behaviors. Some behaviors simply are not acceptable under any circumstance, and you should prohibit these emphatically: "You may not hit another child," "You may not destroy other people's property," or "You may not put other people in danger." Before enforcing proscriptive rules make sure they are essential, for only a handful of behaviors should be absolutely forbidden, and always state them in clear, unequivocal ways. Children often benefit from regular discussion of these guidelines and frequent reminders are critical: "What are the important rules?" "Why do we have these rules?"

Again, efforts to change behavior without substitution usually are unsuccessful or only temporarily helpful. Aggressive behavior is a normal response to frustration. Think about your own response when you feel extremely frustrated and would like to hit the first thing before your eyes. When tension and stress levels rise, many of us have a natural, increased desire to the release these feelings by fulfilling some act of aggression, whether arbitrary or purposeful. As adults we've developed other ways of managing this state of tension, but often it takes very little to overwhelm children with a low tolerance for frustration. For them, an aggressive behavioral response may be the natural reaction.

Frequently frustration results when the child is asked to do something he doesn't want to do (a demand), or forced to stop one activity to transition to another. Schoolwork that is "too difficult," submission to other children who take control, being teased, being punished — all of these situations can result in a state of tension to which the child responds by acting out aggressively.

So what can we offer the child as a substitute for aggression when his state of tension is too high? You can't make a child stop feeling angry, but you can substitute hostile angry behavior with more controlled displays of anger. In fact, just validating the feeling along with setting a limit can be a very powerful intervention: "Derrick, I see that you are feeling very angry, but we cannot hit our friends." Feeling understood and validated often has a calming effect on children (and on adults, too).

Children can manage their frustration by applying the same strategies that adults use: relaxing the tension internally by removing themselves from the situation, talking themselves down, using visualization to imagine a favorite hideaway or activity, counting to ten, closing their eyes, taking a deep breath and letting it out slowly, listening to calming music, or retreating to a place that is soothing. By helping children do these things, you reduce the impulsivity that usually accompanies belligerent behavior. One essential household substitute is a punching pillow or stomping pad, which a child can use when he wants to hurt another child by acting aggressively. Typically, by the time the child has left the site of conflict to go to the stomping corner, he has controlled his impulse and the stomping serves only to release residual tension. Relaxation is incompatible with arousal so if you can help a child to reduce arousal through relaxation, the other more disruptive behaviors that activate the arousal state will begin to languish.

Often people make the case that a child's behavior is an effort to "just get attention," as if the wish to get attention is perverse. In reality, all children need and crave attention; it's simply that children who come from a family situation in which they have been chronically ignored have learned the best way to get attention is through negative behavior. Sometimes these behaviors also may be an effort to gain control. While adults tend to feel manipulated by attention-seeking behaviors, it is more helpful in the problem-solving process to realize the function of such behaviors. Which kinds of behaviors are you ready to provide attention to? How much control are you willing to give a child if she acts appropriately?

Once you discern the function of a behavior, there are many tools at your disposal. Your first step should be to look at the behavior in context and identify a substitute that serves the same function but is socially appropriate. These two measures should serve as guides:

1. Decreasing or eliminating the target behavior.
2. Identifying an appropriate behavior that is incompatible with the target behavior (e.g., relaxation is incompatible with arousal). Although identifying the appropriate behavior generally is not difficult, you must be specific and systematic in your approach.

CASE STUDY: **Tawanda**

You have determined that Tawanda talks most frequently when working on math, her most difficult subject area. Her interruptions occur when she gets excited or when attention is directed away from her. Thus, talking seems to be her way of responding to anxiety, excitement, and lack of attention. Based on this knowledge, what replacement behaviors might you consider?

Case Discussion

Requiring Tawanda to raise her hand when she wishes to speak is one way to help her manage her impulsive need to chatter. Other replacement behaviors for talking to peers or siblings during math or other work, might include a cue Tawanda gives to the teacher that she needs extra help, or pairing her with another child for whom math is an area of strength.

CASE STUDY: **Chris**

Your suspicion regarding Chris's transition problems is supported with baseline information and a conference with his teacher. You discover he discharges excess tension and stimulation when switching from one activity to the next. He also seems to have difficulty structuring his own behavior when there is not a clear, externally imposed structure. Every time there is a switch from spelling practice to vocabulary he gets excited and has trouble calming down. What function could Chris's noisy and disobedient behavior be serving?

Case Discussion

Chris's problematic behaviors serve as his best effort to regulate and structure himself. Understanding that Chris's disobedience is a form of self-regulation, you consider other ways Chris may be able to regulate himself, whether through relaxation, calming strategies, or additional training to enhance his capacity to solve problems and establish structure independently.

STEP 5: **Brainstorm possible interventions**

Once you understand the function of the child's behavior, you
need to generate a list of possible interventions based on substitute
behaviors previously considered. However, in addition to thinking
about the substitute behavior, you need to think about the logistics
of implementing your strategy — what you would use to reinforce
the successful use of the substitute behavior, and how you would
set it up in your home or classroom. For example, if you decide to
set up a "calm-down" corner that a child can use when he feels
overwhelmed and unable to calm herself, be prepared to answer
these questions:

- Where can you set up the calm down corner?
- What resources will you need (e.g., beanbag chair, rug, etc.)?
- How would you help the child use this environment when
  needed?
- How would you reinforce appropriate use of this intervention
  (e.g., reward, points, praise, etc.)?
- How would you explain this intervention to the rest of the
  family?

Examine the possible interventions

Brainstorm several possible interventions, give each serious
consideration, and select the one that makes the most sense and
would be the least intrusive. In making this determination, consider
the potential for effectiveness, the resistance the intervention might
meet, the acceptability and relative intrusiveness to the child, and
the intervention's fidelity as a replacement for the target behavior.

Potential for effectiveness

The first question to be asked is whether the intervention fits both
you and the child. Are you comfortable with the selected plan and
does it address your understanding of the function of the child's

target behavior? Next, does the intervention take into consideration the complexities of the home or school environment? Obviously, every family or classroom has its own limitations and expectations, as well as its own structure. For planned intervention to be effective, you need to be able to implement it within the constraints of your environment. Finally, have you adequately followed the steps in the systematic problem-solving approach so that you know the baseline of the target behavior, the context in which it occurs, and the function it serves? If you can answer these questions, your chosen intervention is much more likely to be effective. The chosen intervention should be

- developed specifically for the behaviors in question,
- appropriate for the situation,
- composed of the proper components,
- administered properly,
- given sufficient time to work (including time for any necessary modifications),
- powerful enough to initiate and maintain change over time.

Acceptability and relative intrusiveness of an intervention

There needs to be a consensus among all the players (both parents, all children, any other members of the family that interact on a steady basis with the child, and, if appropriate, the teacher) that the intervention planned is acceptable and least intrusive as possible. The parent needs to be sure the intervention is compatible with her style, the child needs to "buy into" the plan, and both parents need to agree that a problem exists for which intervention would be advantageous to the child. In the beginning, you may find it helpful to ask others to think through your ideas and design with you, especially experienced colleagues and the school's behavioral specialists. This is likely to increase your own confidence that the planned intervention is a good idea and acceptable to the parties involved.

Resistance and encouragement

For a parent the most significant step toward effective problem solving is the commitment to make changes in yourself and your home. The easiest way to do this is to work with your spouse and other children to improve the home climate. Sometimes you will meet with resistance as you find other parents or teachers who have been beaten down by defeatist attitudes or hold fast to an authoritarian child-rearing style. You may find your spouse is resistant to change and feel frustrated that your efforts are unsupported. Or, if you have leaned toward an authoritarian approach to parenting, you may have to overcome significant obstacles in yourself, battling your own tendencies toward survival and self-interest as your child routinely tests your limits.

Integrity of the intervention

The intervention selected must be fully conceived, executable, and consistently implemented as planned. If you cannot follow through on the plan, then the integrity of the intervention will be significantly compromised and, as a result, almost guaranteed to fail.

Case Study: Tawanda

You want Tawanda to wait her turn to talk at home and during classroom discussions and to ask for help appropriately when she needs it during independent work, especially math. Were she able to do these things, Tawanda would exhibit much better impulse control. What interventions would be appropriate to help Tawanda with her impulsive talking and interrupting?

Case Discussion

After explaining to Tawanda when it is appropriate to talk and when it isn't, you tell her that each time she raises her hand instead of interrupting, she will be given tokens which she can cash in for a treat or toy. You remind her of this goal several times each day and acknowledge her when she waits to talk with you. You let her know that attention will soon be directed her way, if she can wait. Since math assignments create many of the behavioral difficulties for Tawanda, you check with her frequently to make sure she understands the work and can complete it independently. In addition, you encourage her to ask for help when she needs it, and you find a math tutor who can provide extra help in that subject area. If she interrupts or disturbs her siblings while they are trying to do their homework, you isolate her from them and give her a chance to calm herself.

CASE STUDY: **Chris**

You now have a model for thinking about Chris's behavior and some goals to help him learn new ways of self-regulation that will be more adaptive. What interventions would be most effective in helping Chris navigate transitions?

Case Discussion

Chris appears to be typical of many children who have difficulty transitioning from one situation to another. After thinking through the problem-solving process, you realize you have not been properly preparing Chris for transitions; and, while most children adjust to them smoothly, Chris cannot. You develop a routine at home to warn Chris about a transition ten minutes ahead of time; at five minutes you provide a reminder. During transitions, such as preparing for dinner or going out to the car, you keep Chris close to you, putting a hand on his shoulder when you see him begin to lose control. Before any unstructured time at home, you spend a few minutes with Chris, planning what he would like to do. You also want to teach Chris how to manage himself internally through calming strategies such as deep breathing, resting his head on his desk, or leaving an over-stimulating situation instead of relying on others to control him. You talk with Chris's teacher, who agrees to utilize the same intervention strategies.

STEP 6: Communicate interventions to the child

Communication is an important ingredient for a successful intervention and all interested parties need to be fully informed about the plan and given opportunities to contribute and ask questions. To begin with, the intervention must be acceptable to the child, or there is very little chance that appropriate behavior will occur. But the need for acceptability applies at a broader level as well: Is it acceptable to the child's parent, the child's teacher, and the principal? If an intervention is acceptable to all involved parties, then its chance of being successful increases greatly.

Interventions should be regarded as positive both in intent and effect. The child should be included in the process of defining an intervention, since he will be responsible for executing it. In talking with the child as a parent or vested party, you must be nonjudgmental. Begin the conversation by asking questions to understand the child's feelings and to clarify your perceptions of the problem and its function. Then lead the child toward understanding his role in creating the problem by allowing him the opportunity to identify and respond to ideas for a proposed solution. You and the child should work together to set realistic goals and establish ways to evaluate progress.

The child's teacher is an important part of any intervention effort, and it is important to develop a collaborative relationship with him early in the process. If you want the teacher to play a constructive role, you need to remember that the goal is to find solutions to the problem, not someone to blame for it. Once you have developed a plan, invite the teacher to a meeting where the two of you can exchange ideas. Allow him opportunities to question your plan and add any ideas he may have. Create the final plan together, so all the stakeholders can participate and feel ownership in the efforts. The child should be included in at least part of the meeting, so he can see the collaboration between home and school. As you conclude, arrange to have the teacher send you a note or e-mail update each week to keep you apprised of how the intervention is going. Establishing this expectation will confirm a partnership between home and school.

CASE STUDY: **Tawanda**

Now that you've decided on an intervention for the target behaviors, you need to communicate your strategy to Tawanda and her teacher. How do you explain the interventions?

Case Discussion

In a nonjudgmental tone, tell Tawanda that while you understand she is excited and wants to share her thoughts, you disapprove of her interruptions, which disturb both you and her siblings. Let her help you identify a meaningful reward. Attempt to get Tawanda's teacher's support for a reward system at school and communicate with the teacher on a weekly basis in regard to Tawanda's progress.

CASE STUDY: **Chris**

You are now ready to communicate your ideas to Chris and his teacher to allow them opportunities to respond to your ideas and "buy into" these new interventions. What is important in your communication to Chris and his teacher?

Case Discussion

Chris must realize that you believe his behavior is not willful. Help him to understand that sometimes he loses control but there are ways he can learn to keep himself under control. Chris's teacher must be brought into the discussion so he can join in teaching Chris to manage his own behavior more effectively.

STEP 7: **Implement selected interventions**

Implementing the intervention requires planning. By this point you have identified the specific approach you will use, established the logical consequences or reinforcement to be used, and decided how and when to deliver them.

Before you begin implementing the intervention, be sure to ask yourself these questions:
- Do I have all the supplies I will need?
- When will I start?
- How will I evaluate my progress?

With a satisfying set of answers, you are ready to walk the child through the basic features of the intervention:
- Reiterate your plan in simple, positive terms.
- Point out that you believe the child can be successful and that this plan will help things go better at home and in school.
- Be sure to remind the child of what you expect of her.
- Be sure to remind the child of the consequence of her behavior.
- Provide an opportunity for questions. The child needs to feel like a partner in the process and understand how the two of you will work together.

Now, carry out the intervention as planned, keeping in mind some critical rules for yourself:
1. Don't deviate from your goals. You have constructed a plan to address the most problematic behaviors. Minor schoolwork costs that come as a result of developing the child's self-management capacity may be all right for the short run. The real priority you've set will allow the child to make up the work later.
2. Keep your eye on the prize for this child. This may mean the child copies only half the sentences off his homework

assignment or completes only half the math problems. Make sure he does them carefully and accurately.

3. Do not confuse consistency with rigidity. You want the child to be successful because success breeds success, and chronic failure will ensure that your intervention also will fail. The child may need an extra reminder or chance to behave as desired. You may find that your initial plan is too difficult for the child, and you need to lower your expectations so the child can be successful. You can build back up to your original goals over time. Don't back yourself into a corner by declaring your plan as carved in stone. Give yourself some flexibility while remaining consistent in the execution of your stated plan.

4. Use rewards as incentives. Rewards serve as incentives for all of us to exert the extra effort to do something that is genuinely difficult. They help build new capacities in children by encouraging extra effort and serving as enticement for self-management. Some children will respond to verbal praise, others to stickers, others to treats, and others to extra choices. Offering stickers to a child who couldn't care less about them will not give you the "payoff" you seek. Remember for a reward to work, it has to be meaningful to the child. The reward is not the intervention; it is a way to mark success.

5. The name of the game is control. It never feels good to be out of control, neither for children nor adults. Children are frightened by the loss of control but often do not know how to avoid these experiences or regain control after an incident. There is a big, built-in payoff to staying in control—it makes the child feel good.

6. Be empathic. Even as you set limits and manage behavior, you can empathize with a child's experience and emotional state. The child who is frustrated, angry, or overexcited will respond to the feeling that you understand him, even

as you let him know his behavior (e.g., hitting, throwing, running around) is unacceptable. We cannot change the child's feelings, only the way he responds to the feelings. Couch your limit-setting language in empathy: "I see that you are feeling angry, but you may not hit your sister. When you calm down, let's talk about what to do when you feel angry."

7. Be empowering; make sure the child experiences her own success. Remind the child, "I want you to have a good day because it makes you feel good and makes you happy." Offering such reasoning can help the child focus on her internal rewards (i.e., "I feel great about how well I did that!"). The sequence of events becomes aspirational:
   a. The child does what you want her to do
   b. You provide a positive consequence
   c. You enhance her feelings of success, competence, and self-esteem
   d. The likelihood of the child's maintaining the appropriate behavior increases

CASE STUDY: Tawanda

You are now ready to start your new plan to reduce Tawanda's frequent talking and interruptions. What do you need to prepare for implementation?

Case Discussion

There are no special supplies needed for Tawanda other than the tokens and rewards you have selected for reinforcement. You decide to evaluate her progress with the same tools that you used in collecting baseline information. You will remind her each day of the plan, and talk with her for a few minutes at the end of the day about her success or difficulties.

Case Study: **Chris**

Chris's teacher is very enthusiastic about your ideas, and she plans to adapt some of them in her classroom. She also notes that incentives often work for Chris, helping him manage himself. You decide to incorporate incentives into your plan. Are you prepared to implement the selected interventions?

Case Discussion

Helping a child like Chris learn to regulate his own behavior may require a change in your attitude toward Chris and in your parenting style. Try to abandon any notion that Chris is disobedient and "naughty," and understand that his behavior is probably just as distressing for him as you. Commit to changing your parenting style from "being controlling" to "teaching how to control." Post a set of rules and logical consequences that are positive; go over the daily schedule each morning and preview tomorrow's schedule at the end of the day; agree to verbal reminders for prompting him about impending transitions; hold a conference with his teacher to make her aware of Chris's regulatory problems. If the teacher agrees to reinforce your interventions when Chris is in the classroom, follow up with her about Chris's progress. Set up a chart that allows you and Chris to monitor his success each day with special privileges being offered as incentive.

Step 8: **Evaluate and revise interventions**

Give any intervention sufficient time to work, usually at least two weeks. Remember that the target behavior may increase at first; the child is testing to see if you will be consistent and stick with the plan. If the intervention continues without change for two weeks or longer the bad behavior usually will subside, dropping to levels lower than at the start of the intervention. Intervention rarely provokes the target behavior but if it does you may want to make a change before the two-week period is up. Don't forget to remind the child of the plan each day or immediately before a situation that is likely to create a problem.

If the intervention appears successful, evaluating it will not be a problem. Apply the same technique you used to establish the baseline and then compare the results. This comparison can help you explain to the child how the intervention is progressing and can be a source of positive feedback for the child. However, if comparing the data does not indicate success, you will want to make some changes in the intervention. You cannot always predict how a child will react to a new intervention, and you may think of ways to improve your plan:

1. Return to the first step in the problem-solving approach, whether you intend to choose a new intervention or to modify the existing one. Usually, as you review the early steps, you will identify specific issues that require modification, making it easier to adopt appropriate changes.

2. Walk through the whole problem-solving approach as before; repeat the process as many times as needed until you achieve success.

3. If a variety of attempts do not result in success, then you should seek consultation with an experienced professional such as the school counselor or a child psychologist. Consultation is also a good source of support to review interventions that are working effectively and decide when they need modification or should be phased out.

After you've established the amount of progress the child has made, make sure you share information with the teacher. The same things that frustrate parents often frustrate teachers, and hearing about the child's success at home or at school can empower your child's teacher to try different tactics at school, or vice-versa. When parents and teachers support one another and work together, each is less likely to feel criticized for their own struggles in working with a difficult child.

Once the child has mastered a targeted behavior you can begin to phase out the intervention. The intervention may be reduced incrementally so it is not intrusive and rewards or incentives also can be phased out gradually. As rewards are scaled back, children should be encouraged to monitor themselves to determine if they are deserving of the reward and to give themselves the reward for a job well done rather than having it come from an external agent. You might promise a surprise reward at some unexpected time in the future, reminding the child that he needs to maintain the behavior to get a surprise, then once every week or two provide this kind of reinforcement. By this point the child has mastered the new skill and is probably experiencing self-reinforcing payoffs, such as competence, improved relationships, and the feeling of being more in control.

CASE STUDY: **Tawanda**

You have been implementing the intervention for a two-week period. You then spend three days collecting data about the frequency of Tawanda's interruptions and the amount of time she spends talking and disturbing her siblings. After looking at your new data about Tawanda's progress, what revisions would you make in the interventions?

Case Discussion

Reviewing the evaluation data collected over the past few days you feel you have had mixed success. Instances of Tawanda's interrupting and parroting you have decreased slightly. At school her talking has decreased and her math grades have improved. During the first two weeks of the intervention she has waited to talk fifteen times and has collected enough tokens for two special treats. You are not sure how the interventions are going at school because the teacher has not returned your call. You decide that there is enough progress to keep the intervention going, but you think certain areas need modification. You assign an older sibling to be a study buddy who will sit next to her and help her during homework time. You take away time-outs you have used in the past and substitute a reward system.

CASE STUDY: **Chris**

You have been doing all the things you have established as goals in your plan, including talking through calming strategies with Chris when he seems close to losing control. How much progress should you expect to see in Chris during a two-week period?

Case Discussion

Chris has shown little progress in his ability to control the volume of his voice, and only mild improvement transitioning from one activity to another. However there is an immediate positive change in his behavior at the dinner table. Still, despite the hard work you have done to prepare Chris for transitions, the effect is not as great as you had hoped. Teaching self-regulation and control is a long process, and you should not expect to see any great changes in Chris's behavior in two weeks. The important thing is to be consistent and stick to the plan. The more times Chris is prompted and reminded of strategies that will help him stay under his threshold of stimulation, the more he will be able to use those strategies to regulate his behavior. On a brighter note, your success in managing Chris's problems at dinnertime has led you to believe that you are on the right track: he may have difficulty managing space. Because you believe this may be a positive intervention for all your children, you resolve to take steps to make the dinner table less crowded.

The eight-step process described in this chapter is a relatively simple approach to applying behavior management strategies to dysregulated children. However, behavior management alone will not address the emotional and more complex difficulties manifest in alcohol- and drug-exposed children, especially those who have suffered early trauma. In order to address the multifaceted needs of many substance-exposed children, we must incorporate therapeutic interventions from a mental health perspective. This is the subject of the next chapter.

12 Looking for Lord Ganesha

[Lord Ganesha] — the remover of sorrow, the destroyer of obstacles

—John Irving, *Until I Find You*

"When do we give up?" It was a simple question voiced by an overwhelmed adoptive father. After eight years of bouncing around several university health care programs in Chicago, the family had yet to find an answer to Bradley's constant demands, repeated displays of rage, and dangerous threats. The trauma had taken its toll on the entire family, and they were ready to throw in the towel. "We've been to hundreds of lectures and sat through dozens of parenting classes, everything from *1-2-3 Magic* when he was young to behavior modification now. Nothing works. Is it time to give him back to DCFS?"

This father's frustrations had been building for years; the family was in turmoil, and the parents on the verge of divorce. They had reached for every bit of information they could find about alcohol- and drug-exposed children and had done everything in their power to find a therapist for Bradley — some way to manage his behaviors. But it's a bit simplistic for us to think that by understanding the source of behavioral difficulties observed in children, we will be able to solve any problems that may arise. And it is especially simplistic when working with substance-exposed children for whom biologic and environmental factors combine to inform many of the difficulties that we see.

Prevention first

Prior to discussing therapeutic interventions, I need to reiterate the importance of prevention. This is especially true when considering the difficulties of alcohol- and drug- exposed children. Remember, there is a reason for every behavior we see in a child. This may sound rather basic, but no child enjoys being "bad." The question becomes: Can we find the stimulus for the behavior and remove that stimulus?

Presently, we know that a stimulus or "trigger" can come from internal cues or the external environment. As an infant, the child's cues come from biological drives—hunger, thirst, sleep, or anxiety. Later, as the environment becomes more open and complex, external stimuli in the form of the five basic senses—touch, taste, smell, hearing, and vision—emerge as important cues. A loud noise can startle an infant and result in his crying. That same loud noise can startle a school-aged child and pull her off task, leaving her unable to concentrate on the work before her. After administering a test for symptoms, physicians diagnose the child with an attention-deficit disorder, when she simply has trouble screening out unnecessary noises or visual distractions.

Think back to Will, the child introduced in chapter 10, who shouted to the whole class that he had the book *Charlotte's Web* at home. Will's attention kept drifting to the *Charlotte's Web* poster, rather than on the day's lesson about dolphins. Once his tension reached its boiling point, his only release was to shout out in class. The analogy is not all that farfetched: a child exposed to drugs or alcohol prenatally is very much like a pot of water sitting on a stove, always at a simmer—the least stimulus will turn the flame under the pot to full heat, and the water will boil over. One of the most important things we can do to help manage our children's behaviors is to find out what causes the flame to erupt and then work to remove or correct that stimulus from the child's environment. The lesson in Will's case, like the lesson for all substance-exposed children: turn down the heat before the water gets too hot.

If your child is having trouble staying on task when trying to do homework, ask yourself why her attention is being diverted. Look around your child's home study area to see what distractions could be pulling her off task. Rearrange the furniture to create a study corner that is clean, organized, and free from visual distractions. Make sure that the workspace is clutter free, with specific baskets or bins for supplies; and keep study areas clean and plain, avoiding mobiles, hanging items, and other distracting features. Use soft lighting instead of fluorescent lighting, and limit wide-open spaces, perhaps setting up a bookcase to provide a physical boundary for the study area.

You also might consider internal stimuli that may be setting your child off. Are there certain times of day, such as mid-afternoon, when she tends to consistently lose control? Could she be hungry? Would a snack help her stay more regulated? Or is something going on in your family or at school that is making her feel anxious or worried? Children frequently will express such anxiety through temper tantrums that seem completely uncalled for. Talk to your child; find out what might be worrying her. You'll often discover that these worries can easily be addressed through open communication.

Sometimes the easiest solutions are the best solutions, for it is much easier to change the environment, whether external or internal, than to change the child's characteristics, especially when there are changes in the brain due to prenatal exposure to alcohol and drugs. Although it may seem that you are spending a great deal of your time being your child's "external brain," this is what she needs. Your ultimate goal is to shift her away from relying on external controls and help her learn to manage herself.

Some thoughts about therapy

As we begin to address therapy and its manifold expressions, think about how the child acknowledges, interprets, and recognizes stimuli through complex interactions within the brain. From chapter 4 we know that sensory integration deficits are responsible for many of the difficulties a child has in understanding stimuli. Further, prenatal exposure to alcohol, cocaine, tobacco, or other substances can result in structural or functional changes in particular areas of the brain where sensory information is processed. The question now is, "What can be done about it?"

In reality, the behavior we see in the child is her response to a stimulus and to the way that stimulus is organized and processed in the brain. If a child's immediate response is rage, the goal of intervening should be to increase the child's repertoire of possible responses, giving her other ways to respond besides lashing out. However, what often follows the observed behavior is the consequence, either immediate or delayed, in which parents and teachers impose stern pronouncements of what will happen should the child continue to misbehave.

Let us clear up one point right now: delayed consequences have no impact on changing behavior. Many adults recognize the truth of this assertion in their own behavior. As we move into our mid-adult years, many of us make a New Year's resolution to lose weight, believing it is a first step to improved health and longevity. But then we are faced with that chocolate doughnut. We know that if we eat that doughnut, our weight will increase, our cholesterol will go up, our blood pressure will rise, and we may die of a heart attack. Yet what do we most frequently do? We eat the doughnut. The immediate gratification from the taste and texture of that doughnut in our mouth far outweighs the distant consequence of death. In this light, it is easy to understand why warnings such as, "If you don't stop that, Johnny, I'm sending you to your room!" will not control children's behaviors any more than they will alter most adults' behavior.

Thus, our therapeutic approach must encompass a wide range of strategies that can provide children with real preventive alternatives in terms of behavioral self-management. It must understand the structural and functional changes that occur in the brain when a child is prenatally exposed to alcohol or drugs, or when the child suffers early trauma caused by abuse or neglect, family disruption, or inconsistent and multiple placements in a variety of homes. Finally, the approach should account for what parts of the brain have been affected, the age or developmental level of the child, the functioning of the family, and the environment in which the child is living.

A model for treatment

Children with prenatal substance exposure frequently have deficits in self-regulation, socialization, attention, and impulse control. In addition, they struggle to form relationships and often emerge with sensory-processing dysfunction and mood disorders. As a result, when we provide treatment services to these children, our therapy focuses on co-morbid or secondary conditions; we are not "treating" FAS, per se, but its offshoots.

In many cases, it would be easy (but inadvisable) to allow the child's behavior to become the only target, ignoring other important aspects of treatment. Although a clear plan for addressing problematic behavior is necessary, treatment must focus on meeting all of the child's needs, including the child's degree of sensory, emotional, and social development. Appropriate treatment goals and interventions should be multifaceted and approached from several directions simultaneously. This is best facilitated with a model of treatment in which providers from a wide variety of disciplines and training work collaboratively, each bringing his own expertise to bear in addressing the child's needs.

When we discuss multiple disciplines working together, most people, logically enough, automatically envision a "multidisciplinary" approach. However, I advocate for a *transdisciplinary* approach, which calls for much greater interaction and joint participation between parents and providers. First developed by Joseph Shonkoff and his colleagues to provide services to young children with developmental disorders, transdisciplinary implies a "transaction" of ideas and information among professionals and family members. Each professional has a basic theoretical knowledge of the roles, responsibilities and intervention techniques of the other professionals and incorporates treatment aspects of other disciplines into the intervention program. Parents serve as the primary teachers and caregivers and as the central force in the team's goal setting and decision making. This approach empowers the parents in guiding program planning and therapeutic interventions and improves the children's long-term outcome. Children's Research Triangle, almost twenty years ago, conducted a randomized study of foster children who had been prenatally exposed to drugs and alcohol. The outcomes showed that those foster children who participated in transdisciplinary care had fewer placements in the child welfare system, moved to permanency placement more rapidly, and had better developmental outcomes than foster children who received traditional multidisciplinary care. Whatever treatment approach is taken, the children will fare better if team members and parents work together.

Unfortunately, little information exists regarding appropriate treatment approaches for children who have brain-based behavioral, emotional, and cognitive deficits due to a combination of early neglect and prenatal alcohol or drug exposure. Stanley Greenspan, a clinical professor of psychiatry and behavioral science at George Washington University Medical School, offers one notable exception. Throughout his work, Greenspan asserts that the primary goal for children who are at risk for or who are experiencing significant developmental problems is to enable the children to form a sense of their own personhood—a sense of themselves as interactive individuals. That holds true, Greenspan claims, regardless of the source of risk. Optimally, this sense of self is developed within a primary relationship during the early years of an infant's life, so as to facilitate brain growth as well as to support positive mental health. However, for many substance-exposed children, this opportunity does not exist.

Over the past several years at Children's Research Triangle, we have focused much of our effort on developing a model of treatment for substance-exposed children that works to support positive mental health by addressing the early environmental trauma many of these children experience as a result of neglect or abuse. From this work, we have concluded that the therapeutic approach for this population must take into account multiple factors:

1. Children need to be in the presence of their parents—however parents may be defined—so they can be directed toward using the parent for emotional regulation.
2. Parents benefit from assessment of their relationship with their children, so that they can use that information to adjust their interactional patterns.
3. Parents need support and assurance in order to minimize their own anxiety, which can be detrimental to both parents and children.
4. Appropriate psychoeducational instruction helps parents empathize with their child's history and past trauma, decreasing the tendency to "blame" the child for behaviors that are beyond his or her control.
5. Parents must address the way in which they were parented in order to change their own approach to parenting.

Our family-based approach is supported by evidence from a study we conducted of 29 Russian infants adopted out of orphanages by American families. In the study, we analyzed the impact of institutionalization and profound neglect on the quality of attachment and behavioral difficulties in the infant's lives over a period of two years. Our assessment of the children and their adoptive parents found that the strongest correlation with insecure attachment and increased child behavioral difficulties at two years after adoption was not the length of institutionalization and age at adoption but the level of parenting stress documented at the time of adoption. Based on these results, our work in developing treatment programs for young children who have suffered early neglect and who have been prenatally exposed to alcohol or illicit drugs has focused on creating a dyadic model in which parent and child undergo therapy conjointly. The framework for the therapeutic approach is driven by the following theses:

1. Prenatal substance exposure and postnatal neglect detrimentally affect fetal and infant brain growth, producing changes in the structure and function of the limbic system and frontal lobes as well as the prefrontal cortex.

2. The limbic system, frontal lobes, and prefrontal cortex are at the heart of the child's ability to regulate states of arousal and emotions.

3. Dysregulation of arousal and emotions inhibits the young child's ability to respond to and interact with a parent or parent figure.

4. The infant's inability to interact appropriately with the parent interferes with the development of a positive parent-child relationship.

5. It is only within the context of a positive parent-child relationship that normal development occurs.

6. An attuned parent/child relationship will promote development of normal social-emotional functioning, self-control, positive behavior, and long-term mental health in the child.

As shown in Figure 12.1, our therapeutic model integrates education and support for the parent and trauma-informed therapy and sensory integration therapy for the child. The result is a dyadic approach that focuses on improving the relationship between the parent and the child. Within this framework, parents begin to feel more competent and less stress and the child exhibits more appropriate sensory responsiveness as well as enhanced behavioral and emotional regulation. Improvement in these factors leads to better parent/child attunement, since the child's enhanced regulatory capacity allows him to respond more appropriately to the parent, reinforcing the parent's attempts to nurture the child. This mutually reinforcing cycle ultimately leads to improvement in the child's functioning and behavior and paves the way for optimal, long-term mental health outcomes.

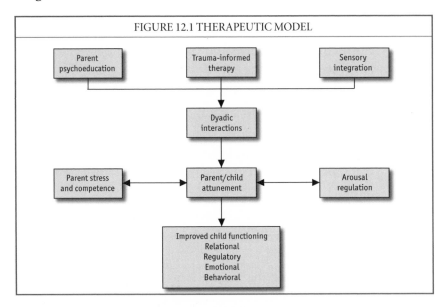

FIGURE 12.1 THERAPEUTIC MODEL

Thinking about therapeutic approaches in this way recognizes that traditional interventions, when used in isolation, may have little effect in working with children who have complex histories. Behavior modification techniques, for example, are often ineffective since prenatal alcohol exposure damages those parts of the brain that allow an individual to associate a consequence with a behavior. Our evidence shows that combining traditional behavior management techniques with hands-on strategies that incorporate multisensory learning, modeling, repetition, and concrete directions within a dyadic context are more effective.

Treatment approaches

Although only a few intervention curricula have been developed to address the specific difficulties faced by children with prenatal alcohol or drug exposure, several programs developed for more general populations or specifically as trauma-informed therapies can be adapted to the needs of alcohol- and drug-exposed children. The following treatment approaches, presented chronologically across a child's life span, are for the most part research-proven and can be melded into our therapeutic model within a transdisciplinary approach. I cannot recommend any one approach over another but wish to emphasize that selection of an appropriate therapeutic intervention should

- directly address the assessed needs of the child, the parents, and the family;
- incorporate a strong psychoeducational component for the parent;
- promote the relationship between the parent and child.

Infants and toddlers

It is well known that among the most important predictors of any child's healthy growth and development is attachment with a consistent, loving parent. Infants and toddlers that are diagnosed with prenatal alcohol exposure often present with severe behavioral dysregulation, speech and language delays, and sensory-processing deficits that disrupt the development of an interactive relationship. Understanding the underlying problems, treating the sensory-processing difficulties, and modifying the environment are critical components of effective treatment. Providing parents with practical methods to help the infant feel secure, such as swaddling, providing periods of quiet time, and creating opportunities for more nurturing caregiving can increase positive interactions. With positive support, the child will be more likely to form secure attachments and coping skills.

The *Developmental, Individual-Difference, Relationship-Based (DIR)* model by Stanley Greenspan and his colleagues is a framework that builds on functional developmental capacities, biologically based processing differences, and emotionally meaningful learning interactions among families, parents, and children. The initial goal is to learn the developmental ("D") level of the child. Therapy accounts for individual ("I") differences in processing in terms of auditory and visual/spatial functioning, sensory modulation, and motor planning. Therapy is delivered in the context of the child's relationships ("R"). Floortime is one component of a comprehensive, DIR intervention program. The approach is simple in its concept—a parent and child squat or kneel on the floor, interacting in a mutually enjoyable encounter. On a broader level, Floortime focuses on creating emotionally meaningful learning interactions that facilitate six functional, developmental capacities in the child: attention, engagement, purposeful emotional signaling and gesturing, preverbal and verbal problem solving, imaginative interactions, and thinking. Other components a DIR-based comprehensive program may include are semi-structured problem solving, learning interactions, speech therapy, occupational therapy, peer play opportunities, and educational programs.

Parent-Infant Psychotherapy (PIP), based on Selma Fraiberg's studies of infants with congenital blindness in the 1970s, focuses on the parent and infant jointly and seeks to improve the relationship between parent and child. When successfully applied the program increases the parents' responsiveness and sensitivity to their child and creates strategies for caregivers to respond to their children's cues in ways that support appropriate development. This model also addresses the unmet emotional needs of the parent, particularly those issues that may impair the caregiver's ability to meet her child's needs. In recent pilot programs, both parents and children showed increased sensitivity, including behavioral and emotional responsiveness, through this type of therapeutic approach.

Preschool-age children

Children with prenatal alcohol or drug exposure often are identified and diagnosed during the preschool years due to problems with general development (i.e., delayed motor or language skills), adaptive tasks, or self-regulation (i.e., distractibility, high level of activity, poor attention). Family-centered, relationship-focused, and dyadic interventions are most effective with this age group.

Parent-Child Interaction Therapy was designed for children 2 to 6 years old with disruptive behavior characteristic of oppositional defiant or conduct disorders, as well as those with insecure attachment. This therapy is intended as a short-term, but not time-limited, intervention (10 to 16 weekly sessions). Emphasis initially is placed on improving the parent-child relationship. Once certain therapeutic goals (i.e., improving the child's obedience and listening, increasing the child's ability to manage frustration and anger, and building the child's self-esteem) have been reached, the emphasis shifts to implementing consistent discipline for the child.

The *Early Childhood Mental Health Dyadic Therapy Program* was developed and piloted at Children's Research Triangle for preschool-age children who have experienced relational, developmental, or behavioral difficulties due to prenatal substance exposure and traumatic histories. The overarching goal is to enhance infant and early childhood mental health, as well as the parent-child relationship, through dyadic group therapy. Over the course of 12 weeks, children receive multisensory interventions intended to improve their ability to respond to positive parenting efforts. Both parents and children are provided with critical information and skills that they can continue to apply in their daily lives. The goals of the dyadic interventions include (1) strengthening the parent-child relationship, (2) guiding parents as they identify reasons for their children's behaviors, (3) supporting parents as they reveal reasons for their own responses to the child, and (4) assisting parents in developing strategies to address concerns they may have with their children. A psychoeducational parent group provides parents with the opportunity to feel understood, supported, and connected with other parents.

Child-Parent Psychotherapy, developed by Alicia Lieberman and Patricia Van Horn, is an empirically validated treatment for children under 6 years. The treatment is flexible and is based in attachment theory but also integrates psychodynamic, developmental, trauma, social learning, and cognitive-behavioral theories. Key components focus on safety; affect regulation; improving the child-caregiver relationship; normalization of trauma-related responses; and joint construction of a trauma narrative, with the goal of returning the child to a normal developmental trajectory.

School-age children

School-age children or adolescents with prenatal exposure may demonstrate deficits over multiple domains, including executive functioning, sensory integration, self-regulation, and interpersonal relationships. Challenges in these areas put the children and older youth at high risk for experiencing low self-esteem, mood disorders, and isolation from peers. There is a wide range of effective therapeutic interventions for children 7 to 17 years old. However, because children with prenatal substance exposure are more susceptible to a wide variety of co-morbid mental health problems that must be addressed concurrently, identifying appropriate treatment approaches can be challenging.

Dyadic Developmental Psychotherapy (DDP) was developed by the clinical psychologist Daniel Hughes to address trauma-based attachment problems in children with complex histories. DDP is based on the theory that the parent-child relationship greatly influences the development of the child. Treatment and parenting interventions facilitate security and incorporate an attitude based on playfulness, acceptance, curiosity, and empathy. Parents are educated about their child's emotional needs and about the way the child's thinking processes work. They are then instructed in parenting strategies that promote safe and appropriate management of behaviors. The therapist models for the parent crucial ways of engaging the child, frequently alternating throughout the session between the therapist-child relationship and the parent-child relationship.

Cognitive Behavioral Therapy (CBT) has been found most effective in treating children with mood disorders, commonly found among children with prenatal alcohol and drug exposure. The principles of CBT and its use with children have been well defined in a number of publications. CBT provides effective symptom relief for a wide range of mood, anxiety, attention, self-regulation, and behavioral disorders. A child's self-esteem and competence grow as he learns and practices new skills and problem-solving strategies. Integrating sensory-based and experiential interventions is recommended with children that may have neurocognitive deficits due to prenatal substance exposure or complex trauma. It is important to make adaptations, such as integrating play-based approaches into traditional CBT, in order to meet the child's developmental level and capabilities.

Project Brain Buddies, developed by Mary O'Connor and her colleagues at the University of California at Los Angeles, is a social skills training program that aims to improve peer friendships for children with fetal alcohol spectrum disorders. Designed for children 6 through 12 years old, the intervention and its social skills components are based on the developmental psychology literature pertaining to children's friendships. Children participate in 12 sessions, 90 minutes in length, delivered over the course of 12 weeks. Parents attend separate, concurrent sessions in which they receive education on the features of FASD and are instructed on key social skills being taught to their children. Published research has revealed significant improvement in children's knowledge of appropriate social behavior and use of social skills, and a decrease in the appearance of problem behaviors, when this program is used. These improvements were maintained over a 3-month period.

The *Math Interactive Learning Experience (MILE)* designed by the clinical psychologist Claire Coles and her colleagues at the Marcus Institute of Emory University aims to improve the behavioral and math functioning of alcohol-affected children 3 through 10 years of age. The psychoeducational program provides learning strategies to compensate for core alcohol-related neurodevelopmental deficits; it includes intensive, short-term, individual instruction for the child as well as training for caregivers and teachers. The goal is to provide a consistent method of mathematical instruction across therapeutic, home, and school environments, through 6 weeks of tutoring services with the child. Caregivers receive instruction in supporting math learning at home and are given weekly home assignments to complement the individualized tutoring sessions. Caregiver education, case management services, and psychiatric consultations are included. All children and their families receive standard psychoeducational treatment, which consists of a comprehensive neurodevelopmental evaluation, assistance with educational placement, and development of the child's individualized educational plan.

Families Moving Forward (FMF) was developed at the University of Washington under the leadership of Susan Astley and Heather Carmichael-Olson. Specific goals of the program are to improve caregiver self-efficacy, meet family needs, and reduce problem behaviors in children with FASD by modifying parenting attitudes and parenting responses toward the child's problem behaviors. Designed for children 5 to 11 years old and their caregivers, the FMF intervention is a low-intensity, sustained model of supportive behavioral consultation. The program lasts 9 to 11 months, including at least 16 biweekly, 90-minute sessions. Limited and focused consultation to school staff and community providers are available, and intervention providers work to link families to needed resources in the community.

Neurocognitive Habilitation Therapy is a treatment approach developed over the past eight years at Children's Research

Triangle. As we attempted to translate our knowledge of prenatal substance exposure into a practical approach to therapy, we conceptualized the children's difficulties as prenatal brain injury and incorporated treatment strategies for pediatric traumatic brain injury (TBI). When anyone suffers trauma to the brain, the frontal lobe frequently sustains substantial injury due to its large size. Frontal lobe dysfunction results in decreased judgment and increased impulsivity, irritability, aggression, and socially problematic behaviors. These behaviors, of course, are consistent with clinical findings within the population of children affected by prenatal exposure to alcohol and drugs.

As discussed previously, many of the maladaptive behaviors commonly observed in children with substance exposure have origins in dysregulated levels of arousal. In order to address the children's ability to self-monitor and ultimately self-regulate, thereby improving the capacity for executive functioning, we also incorporate components of arousal therapy as described in the *Alert Program*, developed by two occupational therapists, Mary Sue Williams and Sherry Shellenberger. Our goal is to teach parents (and children) to monitor, maintain, and change the child's level of alertness as appropriate to a situation or task.

The program consists of a 12-week curriculum for children 6 to 12 years old with prenatal alcohol and drug exposure and for their families. Caregiver and child groups are conducted concurrently and last approximately 75 minutes; the final 15 to 30 minutes provide an opportunity for parents and children to come together to practice what they learned during that week's session.

Neurocognitive Habilitation Therapy teaches children awareness of their body states and arousal levels. Once children are able to accurately identify arousal levels, they learn strategies to maintain an alert, relaxed state. This may be achieved by calming themselves if they are overactive and fidgety, or arousing themselves if they are tired or "down." Throughout the 12-week curriculum, concepts related to self-esteem, sequencing of tasks, cause-and-effect reasoning, problem solving, and emotional awareness are introduced. Parents learn to promote their children's self-regulation abilities, while children work toward improving their executive functioning skills.

Adolescence

Many children with prenatal alcohol and drug exposure present with complex and chronic symptomatology due to a history of chaotic relationships and physical or emotional trauma. The *Attachment, Self-Regulation, and Competency (ARC)* framework, designed for youth from early childhood through adolescence, provides a theoretical foundation, core principles of intervention, and a guiding structure for providers working with traumatized children and their caregivers. Preliminary data from pilot studies indicate that ARC leads to reduction in child posttraumatic stress symptoms, anxiety, and depression, and increases adaptive and social skills. Parents often report reduced distress and view their children's behaviors as less dysfunctional.

Structured Psychotherapy for Adolescents Responding to Chronic Stress (SPARCS) is a predominantly cognitive-behavioral group intervention that was designed to address the needs of adolescents with complex histories who are living with ongoing stress and are experiencing problems in several areas of functioning. These areas include difficulties with affect regulation and impulsivity, self-perception, relationships, dissociation, numbing and avoidance, physical ailments and struggles with their own purpose and meaning in life. Overall goals of the program are to help teens cope more effectively in the moment, enhance self-efficacy, connect with others, and establish supportive relationships.

Medication treatment

A full discussion of the various medications that have been used to treat the many co-occurring mental health disorders that may be present in substance-exposed children is beyond the scope of this book. However, as discussed in chapter 6, the majority of these children exhibit behaviors consistent with a diagnosis of ADHD. We therefore will briefly address the use of stimulant medications for children prenatally exposed to alcohol and illicit drugs.

There is no question that medication treatment of children with classic, genetic ADHD is beneficial. The American Academy of Pediatrics indicates that for many children with ADHD, the best way to mitigate symptoms is though the use of a combined approach to intervention that integrates behavior management and medication. This method, referred to in the literature as "multimodal" treatment, has been shown to improve academic performance, parent-child interaction, and school-related behaviors. It also has been found to reduce childhood anxiety and oppositional behaviors. Several longitudinal studies have shown that children who require medication but do not receive it are more likely to use illegal drugs when they are older than children who are placed on appropriate stimulant medications. However, the decision as to whether to treat a child with medication or not is a complex and difficult one. Above all, appropriate intervention and treatment planning must begin by the physician's looking beyond observable behaviors to try to understand the biological and emotional sources of those behaviors.

Until recently, there has been little understanding as to how common ADHD drugs, such as Ritalin, work. Doctors have continued to prescribe these stimulants in large numbers, however, for the simple reason that in many cases they do indeed work. A recent study from the University of Wisconsin, Madison, examined the effect of ADHD drugs on the brain. The researchers reported that stimulant drugs primarily target the prefrontal cortex, the regulatory center in the front of the brain associated with attention, decision making, and an individual's expression of personality. The stimulant medications evaluated in the study boosted levels of two chemical messengers—dopamine and norepinephrine. As discussed previously, these neurotransmitters are linked to memory formation, arousal, and attentiveness. Working with rats, the researchers conducted laboratory and behavioral tests to ensure that animal drug doses were functionally equivalent to doses prescribed in humans. Afterwards the research team measured concentrations of dopamine and norepinephrine, in three different brain areas, in the presence and absence of low-dose stimulant medication. Under the influence of stimulants, dopamine and norepinephrine levels increased in the rats' prefrontal cortex. This appears to be the reason stimulant drugs, such as Ritalin, Concerta, Adderall and other similar compounds, improve behavior in many children with classic ADHD or ADD.

However, while numerous studies have examined the effectiveness of stimulant treatment on school-aged children, there is little information regarding the use of these medications in preschool-aged children. There are important reasons why the results from treatment studies are not applicable at this age. The developing nervous system of preschoolers is less organized than that of older children. In addition, because preschoolers lack the reasoning skills, social development, and academic skills of school-aged children, interventions successful with older children may be ineffective at this age. On the other hand, failing to treat ADHD in very young children may compromise their safety, since attention and behavior problems often begin before children start kindergarten. Moreover, research has demonstrated that very young children with ADHD are at risk for school failure; and without early intervention, their behavioral problems may worsen when they reach the academic challenges of elementary school.

To date, several reviews of studies evaluating medication treatment for young children with ADHD have been conducted. An examination of nine controlled studies concluded that stimulant treatment largely was found to be beneficial in treating preschoolers with ADHD. Another review of pertinent research concluded that stimulants can improve compliance, on-task behavior, and activity levels in young children with inattention, impulsivity, and hyperactivity. However, there are serious limitations in these studies:

- Lack of comparison children who do not receive medication so that the researchers can consider all other influences on outcome
- Small numbers of children enrolled in the studies
- Short duration of stimulant medication trials without any long-term follow-up of the children
- Inconsistent criteria as to which children were eligible for the studies
- Too much reliance on parent and teacher reports without the corroboration of laboratory psychological tests

Despite the lack of solid research information to guide clinicians, stimulant treatment for preschoolers is becoming more and more common. In a 2002 study, a group of researchers examined the patterns of medication used in children 3 years old and younger with symptoms consistent with ADHD. Of 223 children studied, 57% were receiving pharmacological treatment. However, the medications were being prescribed in an erratic and inconsistent manner: a total of 22 different medications were being used, in 30 different combinations, in this very young population of children.

Research on the use of stimulant medications in older, school-age children has fared better. It is clear that the use of these medications benefits many children, and medication clearly is indicated in a number of substance-exposed children. Certainly, our role as clinicians is to ensure that children who will benefit from medication do receive it in an appropriate dose and with close monitoring. Yet proper diagnosis takes time — I do not consider medication interventions until a thorough evaluation has been completed and behavioral interventions have been implemented. Without such an approach, the family falls into the trap of relying on medication as the primary intervention rather than following through with behavioral management strategies that should really be the first step. Thus, the decision to use medication should be made only *after* behavioral interventions have been instituted and within the context of a team meeting. Parents and the clinical team should reach consensus on the treatment approach and jointly develop a monitoring plan that includes active involvement from the child, family, and school.

Compassion fatigue

Parents, teachers, and other caregivers who work with traumatized and substance-exposed children often find themselves in a bind because of the overwhelming stress of working with affected children day in and day out. This is the risk we endure when engaging empathically with a traumatized child. Our energy is depleted, we feel a wide range of emotions, we vascaillate from anger to sadness, from anxiety to rage. The ongoing stress can disrupt our frame of reference so that our very sense of self is disrupted. We may shut down emotionally, withdraw from social activities, and be unable to meet our own psychological and relational needs. Ultimately, we lose our ability to respond to the child in an empathic, caring, and compassionate manner.

We become the victim.

This is a very human response, but we have to remember that our children depend on us. When the situation begins to look grim, recognize the great resiliency that children seem to have and tune in to the positive aspects of helping young people heal. Stay connected to the present, keep the big picture in view, join a group of parents like you who are raising substance-exposed and traumatized children. Most of all, realize that every step you take with a substance-exposed, traumatized child is a step toward that child's healing and health. And remember, as parents, caregivers, and teachers, we have to keep our sense of humor. We may not find Lord Ganesha, but we can find the right balance of behavior management and mental health interventions to help our children fulfill their potential for a healthy life.

PART IV
THE POLITICS OF POLICY

13 The GoodEnough Syndrome

Stand ten feet away from a wall. Now walk halfway to the wall and stop. Continue in this manner, walking half the distance each time you move forward. As you advance you'll see the wall coming closer, you may even be able to touch it. But you'll never make it all the way to the wall.[1]

This dilemma is a good illustration of what I have come to call the GoodEnough Syndrome: a mindset of moving forward inch by inch without ever making progress, a pattern of thinking that sedates like an opiate, convincing us that going half-way is "good enough." In this sense, the GoodEnough Syndrome is characterized by policies and practices that use the lowest common denominator of achievement to define success—usually financial or political success rather than human success.

The truth is we are falling short. The GoodEnough Syndrome's failure to improve the lives of children occurs for many reasons, but above all it comes from a lack of conviction. When it is time to sit down and discuss policy, lawmakers are willing to acquiesce for the sake of diplomacy and compromise. This social phenomenon was explained in 1974 by Jerry Harvey, the professor emeritus of management science at George Washington University, as the Abilene paradox. It occurs in organizations in which agreement is

---

[1] This scenario was first presented by the philosopher Zeno and later expanded upon by Aristotle as an argument against pluralism—the belief in the simultaneous existence of many things rather than one. Zeno was defending Parmenides of Elea, a Greek philosopher from 5th century BCE, against critics who rejected his singular view of reality.

reached and action is taken despite the fact that each individual in the group, if polled privately, would say the result is something he does not desire (think about the various federal health care reform bills recently under consideration by Congress). Best intentions lie behind most examples of the GoodEnough Syndrome. But multiple forces grounded in political and economic realities elbow their way to the front of the room, dilute the best intentions, and drive us toward that lowest common denominator through which we can claim success.

TABLE 13.1 POLICIES AND PRACTICES OF THE GOODENOUGH SYNDROME
• Reactive rather than proactive
• Grounded in terms of financial rather than human cost
• Focus on singular problems or diagnoses rather than co-occurring disorders
• Determine service access based on eligibility rather than need
• Restrict range, intensity, and duration of services
• Define success in terms of broad quantitative measures geared to participation and contact rather than client-oriented outcomes
• Designed *within* systems rather than *across* systems
• Allow *service* integration to substitute for *systems* integration

Political pressure plays no small role, and even well-intentioned bills fall prey to the effacing effects of compromise. On June 25, 2003, President George W. Bush signed the Keeping Children and Families Safe Act, reauthorizing the Child Abuse Prevention and Treatment Act (CAPTA). Within this reauthorization are a number of additions to the eligibility requirements states have to fulfill in order to receive their federal share of child abuse prevention money. Among these additions, one stands out: the requirement that hospitals and all health care personnel report any child to the state's child welfare system if the child is born "affected" by maternal use of illegal drugs during pregnancy or exhibits withdrawal symptoms resulting from prenatal drug exposure. The child welfare system is then responsible for developing a "plan of safe care" for every reported drug-exposed infant and referring these children to early intervention services for infants and toddlers with disabilities. At first glance the program, funded through Part C of the 2004 federal Individuals with Disabilities Education Act (IDEA), appears to be a good idea.

But what is the reality? The intended goal of the legislation was to develop a system that ensured all children born at risk due to maternal substance abuse would have access to early intervention services. Morally, no one could argue with the bill's intent. Voting against it would be to forever to wear the slur "anti-child" and "pro-drug abuse." The legislation passed easily. However, no funds were made available to institute training for hospitals and health care personnel on how to recognize a substance-exposed child. Worse, it was unclear what the term "affected" really meant. Did a positive urine toxicology qualify a child as "affected?" Finally, where was alcohol in the legislation? Although alcohol is the leading cause of disabilities among this population of children, the bill specifically excluded prenatal alcohol exposure as a condition for referral. In light of what is known in the scientific community about the health and developmental risks alcohol poses to these children, passage of the bill can only be seen as the result of a crisis of confidence. Stakeholders cowed when it came time to settle on the bill's final language. Critics speculated that economic interests of the beer, wine, and liquor industries unduly influenced the CAPTA legislation. And undoubtedly, the presence of a robust alcohol lobby is antithetical to a healthy discourse about the proper course of intervention for alcohol-exposed children.

CAPTA is just one of many examples of how economic pressure can stifle programs for children at risk. The 2009 economic downturn brought a rash of GoodEnough decisions, not the least of which was dismantling the social service systems in many states. For decades many California counties' mental health crisis centers provided immediate access to individuals with an acute mental health emergency. With a simple telephone call, families in need were able to access assessment, treatment, and institutionalization, on an emergent basis. However, as funding in the state dwindled, these crisis centers were among the first to be dismantled. Now, in some California counties, if a citizen calls the mental health crisis center, the recorded message advises the family to go to the emergency room — a visit that costs many times more than entrance into the mental health system through a crisis center and is much more intimidating and threatening for someone in the midst of a mental health emergency.

The abstract child

Language is the foremost tool of the GoodEnough Syndrome. Images and labels provide a framework for contemplation and communication. For example, the word "circus" brings to mind performances in three rings, spotlighted thrills — a tent filled with laughing and applauding children; we do not "see" the word circus but the pictures it evokes. In the case of the GoodEnough Syndrome, language is used to summon dark and sinister images. The abundant use of the phrase "crack baby" in the 1980s, for instance, cemented in the popular imagination the image of a tremulous, seizing baby, abandoned in his bassinet by his drug-addicted mother living on the fringe of society. The knee-jerk response of many states was to create laws that punished the mothers. This was easy to do since the media's portrayal of crack using pregnant woman, in general, was African American, inner city women, who, because of their own moral lethargy, didn't deserve to have children anyway. As long as society could mythologize substance abuse in the language of "them" vs. "us," the children and families remained enigmatic. As a society, we would "rescue" the babies, throw their mothers in jail, and sleep well at night. This was *good enough.*

The media have had their hand in this injustice. As we saw in the 1980s, attempts to clearly define the difficulties that drug-exposed babies display frequently are distorted when seen through the lens of the media. Immediately after reports of normal cognitive functioning in cocaine-exposed children emerged in the scientific community, there was a swing in how the issue was presented in the nation's newspapers. Suddenly, news outlets were reporting that prenatal cocaine exposure had no impact on child outcome. This pendulum of contradictory information guaranteed children would remain an abstract illusion of small advocacy groups on one side of the question or the other. As a nation, we very adroitly developed policies to punish in the guise of protection, rather than policies that would support improved family functioning and child outcomes.

Deficit labeling

We use words that simplify the problem of substance use for convenience and accessibility. Even though we now have a wealth of data that describes both the strengths and weaknesses of children prenatally exposed to cocaine, methamphetamine, heroin, and a variety of other "hard" drugs, our language tends to focus on the weaknesses. It is much easier to connect emotionally to a mental picture of the fragile, tremulous child who has been harmed by his mother's drug use than to the child who is relatively healthy and thriving because of early intervention. Prevention has no meaning in the hard vernacular of politics.

Deficit labeling is nothing new. It dates back to the 1950s, when anthropologist Oscar Lewis, writing of a "culture of poverty," claimed that the poor belong to a special culture that has existed in poverty for so long they have adapted to its characteristic features. According to Lewis, many of the poor are burdened by a sense of helplessness and dependency and have no desire to escape the conditions in which they live. Echoes of this view can be heard today. Following Hurricane Katrina in 2005, Barbara Bush, touring the Astrodome where many of the poorest citizens of New Orleans were being warehoused, observed, "What I'm hearing, which is sort of scary, is that they all want to stay in Texas. Everybody is so overwhelmed by the hospitality. And so many of the people in the arena here, you know, were underprivileged anyway so this [chuckle]—this is working very well for them." The former first lady expresses the skepticism abounding in this country regarding the intentions of the poor. The undertone is that the victims of Hurricane Katrina are morally deficient, unworthy of our help. We see this attitude reflected in the punitive approaches several states have adopted in response to pregnant women who use drugs. Addiction is a matter of will power, so the thinking goes, and if the women really wanted to stop using they would. This attitude, in addition to reinforcing dangerous stigmas, ignores the scientific reality that addiction is a chronic, relapsing disease, not a moral failing.

Labeling and diagnosis

Access to medical and psychological services also is grounded in labels, though instead of using terms such as "underprivileged," we refer to children based on "diagnoses." He's bipolar, or she's ADHD. The absurdity of how we typically use these labels becomes clear when we consider referring to diseases this way: she's cancer, or he's Parkinson's. However the fact remains that in most states, in order for a child to receive eligibility and reimbursement for early mental health services, the child must receive a diagnosis based on clinical labels outlined in *DSM-IV*. Although this label may serve as a necessary form of classification, it also stigmatizes a child and in fact may lead to a self-fulfilling prophecy, especially when the child is consistently viewed through the prism of the diagnosis.

Think back to chapter 6 when we discussed Alex, the three-year-old child with emotional dysregulation resulting from alcohol-induced changes in the corpus callosum. You'll recall that Alex was experiencing "rages" without any precipitating event; his emotions were labile and unpredictable. Numerous children like this are referred to Children's Research Triangle with a diagnosis of bipolar disorder; yet the criteria for this diagnosis were created for adults. Assigning these diagnostic labels to preschoolers qualifies the children for mental health services but risks driving the child toward inappropriate medication. More often than not, children like Alex already are on powerful, anti-psychotic medication when they arrive at our clinic. Here again, a prime example of The GoodEnough Syndrome: we have made the child eligible for services, but at the cost of inappropriate treatment.

I propose we move away from requiring *DSM-IV* diagnoses for the treatment of young children and talk more in terms of "functional diagnoses." By functional diagnosis, I mean utilizing diagnostic terms that clearly describe a child's behavior and consequently drive treatment planning and service delivery. A few states currently have moved to such a system. Expanding on Stanley Greenspan's *DC: 0-3* diagnostic codes for children birth to three years of age, these states grant Medicaid reimbursement and service access to all children through five years of age who meet criteria for a functional diagnosis. In the past, "bipolar disorder" was simply the most convenient diagnosis that would allow Alex to receive services. Now he would receive a diagnosis of "emotional dysregulation," directing a course of treatment based on sensory integration, dyadic, and developmental therapy rather than medication. In addition, we move away from a term like "bipolar" that implies, however subtly, that this child is unteachable and unredeemable, a child for whom no amount of money or effort will make a difference. I recognize that a move toward functional diagnoses will be a difficult one, since the use of *DSM* criteria and special education categories are so deeply ingrained in institutional practices. However, progress is being made, and the *DSM-V*, currently under discussion and review, does contain a new diagnostic category, "behavioral dysregulation." A potential victory for young children.

The politics of service access

The movement toward functional diagnoses is important for another reason. It illustrates how vital government funding is as a policy instrument to guide access to a variety of services, including early intervention and educational programming. Funding granted through IDEA is an expression of the political will that all children with early developmental delays should have access to early intervention services. IDEA mandates that children birth to three years of age receive services if they meet specific criteria including documented developmental delays or a medical diagnosis associated with developmental delays (such as Down syndrome). The third set of criteria to guide eligibility, "demonstration of risk for developmental delays from environmental or other factors," is left for each state to define.

Although the legislation appears to be a step in the right direction, the problem lies in the narrow definition of eligibility under which children are granted services. A review of current policies across states reveals guidelines that define access based on eligibility rather than need, restrictions that limit the range of services provided, and therapeutic choices that selectively serve economic rather than client ends. Despite good intentions, we have created a machinery of neglect that serves some children well but leaves the great majority to fend for themselves. Children with minor speech and language delays, for example, do not qualify for services until the untreated speech difficulties become worse or begin to affect other areas of development. Thus, we focus our resources on children who are in the worst shape, and who, as a result, probably will have a less successful response to services provided. Of course, severely affected children need services and should receive them; but, by taking such an all or nothing approach, we eliminate opportunities for children with milder problems who need services and likely would benefit the most from them.

GoodEnough economics

There is no eluding the fact that economic realities drive health care and social services policy decisions. Programs must be driven by results. They must be affordable. Nevertheless, in making these decisions, policy makers perpetuate the GoodEnough Syndrome by using economic data that are limited in scope and demonstrate a lack of understanding of the family dynamic lying at the core of economic hardship. For children exposed to alcohol and other drugs during pregnancy, the most commonly applied economic data examine state and national costs for treating fetal alcohol syndrome (FAS). Data focus on health-related factors: the costs of care for low birth weight infants, surgical correction of alcohol-related birth defects, heart defects, and auditory defects, and care for moderate or severe mental retardation. Since 1980 there have been multiple studies of the annual cost for FAS, ranging from $250 million to $3.2 billion.

However, what is missing in all of these studies is the out-of-pocket cost foster and adoptive parents take on in caring for a child who falls into the broader spectrum of deficits produced by prenatal alcohol exposure. These families often lack the financial resources and support to ensure the child's access to services, yet are excluded from programs because their child does not meet stringent eligibility criteria. Children with FAS and mental retardation receive services; children with alcohol-related neurodevelopmental deficits (ARND) most often do not. No economic studies directly address the variability in diagnosis that occurs across the fetal alcohol spectrum, the sequence of treatment for the organic anomalies associated with ARND, the psychological and behavioral costs associated with ARND, the quality of life of individuals with ARND, the effect of the family environment on the child with ARND, the progression and treatment of ARND over time, or the accessibility of community services for diagnosing FAS and ARND. Most important, while existing studies focus on societal, health care, provider, and payer costs, none collect data to address the full range of costs to the families who are raising these children.

The financial support provided to foster and adoptive parents who are raising children with FAS and ARND varies widely across the states but falls consistently below the cost of raising a child with no problems. For example, the U.S. Department of Agriculture estimated the average cost of raising a healthy nine-year-old child, excluding medical care, was $8,260 per year in 2000. However, during that same period, the average amount provided to foster parents to meet the needs of a healthy nine-year-old child was $4,932 per year—about half the cost required to raise a child who has no cognitive or behavioral disabilities. In Illinois, this rate can be enhanced depending on the child's age, the child's special needs, the foster parent's training and experience, or emergency status, but still remains below actual costs. These low rates of reimbursement stand in stark contrast to state child welfare agencies' concerns regarding foster and adoptive parent recruitment and retention. Expenses related to recruiting and training parents and the psychological cost of foster parent turnover to a vulnerable child magnify the problem. Although adoption subsidies are available in many states, many adoptive parents do not know to request such long-term support.

These issues are complicated by the fact that families often do not know they are adopting a special needs child who has been prenatally exposed to alcohol or drugs. But as the exposed child grows older, psychological problems complicate the biologically based cognitive deficits, resulting in a variety of behavioral problems and emotional disturbances that could not have been predicted when the adoption subsidy was being formulated. Likewise, social relations present increasing challenges for the alcohol-exposed child. Commonly, family members share the social costs of alcohol- and drug-exposed children through the emotional pain and isolation associated with raising a child with special needs.

The complexity of prenatal exposure makes economic modeling extremely difficult. As a starting point, though, I put forth a bio-psychosocial representation of the economic costs of fetal alcohol spectrum disorders (FASD), designed to capture the full spectrum of alcohol exposure as well as the full spectrum of the family's economic burden. At its heart the model considers three key questions: (1) *Who should be factored into a cost model?* (2) *Who bears the greatest cost?* and (3) *How do we assess costs accurately and precisely?*

In Figure 13.1, the provider is at the center because this is where all the money ultimately gets funneled. The family overlaps all payor levels since the cost of caring for the child is ultimately the family's responsibility.

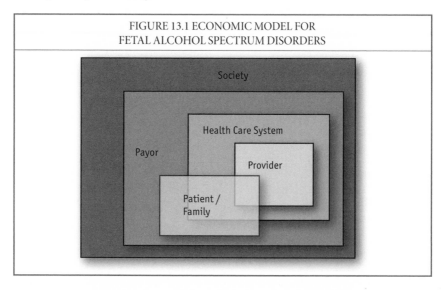

FIGURE 13.1 ECONOMIC MODEL FOR
FETAL ALCOHOL SPECTRUM DISORDERS

As the model is constructed, there needs to be a high degree of precision in defining what constitutes cost. Under current methods of cost analysis, costs for society, insurance companies, the health care system, and the provider are the primary considerations. Although the family is most affected by the costs of raising a child with FASD, what those family costs are remains a distant concern. By reversing this usual strategy and approaching cost analysis from a family perspective, we are able to address indirect and intangible costs that usually are lost. These hidden costs include the emotional costs and lifestyle adjustments that accompany raising a child with FASD. Thus, the bio-psychosocial model of economic burden addresses family costs across three domains that overlay societal, payor, health care system, and provider costs:

- **Direct costs** This is the category of costs most commonly considered when addressing the economic burden of a particular disease entity; namely, those costs directly associated with paying for interventions or treatment strategies required by the child with FASD. An important consideration in measuring direct costs is the source of payment. While some direct costs are paid directly by the family, others are paid by outside parties such as insurance companies and state welfare agencies. Thus, in most cases, there will be a difference between the services a family uses and those they actually pay for. While both types of expenses need to be considered, there never has been a focus on the family's out-of-pocket expenditures. This is a necessity if we are to acknowledge that many families must seek services that are not funded through the usual payor systems.

- **Indirect costs** These costs, attributed to the child's treatment but incurred as a result of obtaining auxiliary services or because of the increased strain on family functioning, place a significant burden on the family. They have never been measured. Most notably, productivity losses attributable to caring for the child result in a decrease in production and income for one or both parents and can encompass a broad range of costs, including days of work lost, family disruption, changes in work patterns, changes in leisure time, and additional expenses such as the cost for family therapy.

- **Intangible costs** Families raising a child with FASD suffer a wide range of intangible costs, which comprise a much less quantifiable subset of indirect costs. Intangible costs account for non-material losses for the families: anxiety, fear, pain, suffering, social isolation, to name a few.

Unfortunately, it is unlikely that the comprehensive studies needed to understand family costs will ever be undertaken. It is *good enough* to bemoan societal and payor costs for FASD. Exposing the economic reality of the cost of FASD to families would force child welfare systems to increase support to the families. In fact, when such a study was proposed to the Illinois Department of Children and Family Services, the former director refused to sign off, stating, "If we know what it costs to raise a child like this, then we'll have to pay foster parents enough to take the children in. We can't afford it."

Expediency

The political dynamics of the GoodEnough Syndrome demand we choose only two from among three core elements for effective early intervention: good, fast, and cheap. As providers, we of course seek programs that are good and fast, programs that impact children in a positive manner within a short time frame. However, those kinds of programs are very expensive. If we turn to fast and cheap, it is doubtful that any good will be accomplished. Good and cheap might work, but the program necessarily will be conducted in a very focused manner, limited to very few children. With this approach, meeting the needs of all the children with prenatal substance exposure — or any type of developmental delays — is impossible.

Instead of this pick-and-choose approach, what is desperately needed is a viable, sustainable set of policies and practices that combine moral decision making based on how we want the world to work, economic reality as to how the world does work, and scientific thinking that puts into practice effective and proven strategies to deliver the highest quality of care. Within such an approach, family-based prevention and early intervention become an economic as well as a moral obligation.

Recognizing the GoodEnough Syndrome

The GoodEnough Syndrome lurks behind every piece of state and federal legislation. As an advocate for children, watch out for oversimplified data crunching: policies and programs come and go, but rarely are they clearly evaluated. Federal and state programs, in particular, are notorious for relying on quantitative rather than qualitative outcome to define success. Evaluation is geared toward quantifying participation and contact, rather than asking meaningful questions that indicate if the child is actually getting better.

Beware the myth of sustainability. No matter how successful a program may be on the site level, the fact is that grant-funded projects are not easily generalized to a community. The small population of participants, the low staff-to-child ratio, and the constantly changing demographic, social, and economic conditions challenge successful evolution of these programs to institutionalization within the community. Nevertheless, requirements for "sustainability" are tossed around; project officers assure grantees that if their program is successful, other funds will become available through existing funding streams such as Medicaid. This simply is not true. Rather, it is the funding agencies' way of saying, "We've done what we can. It's time for us to move on to the next problem." In other words, "Our funding your start up is 'good enough.' Now these kids are your problem."

Watch out for policies marked by ethical sleight-of-hand, those that diminish the impact of a program on children by appropriating resources toward competing demands. This is especially true when demands are driven by pork-barrel politics. Despite enticing political promises, the net impact of Illinois lottery dollars for education was minimal because for each lottery-generated dollar given to education, a dollar was siphoned off to support another arm of the state budget. And of course there is the classic property tax funding scheme, well described in several works by Jonathon Kozol, in which the poorest children go to the most poorly financed and lowest functioning schools. Finally, my favorite—the "any body is better than no body," stonewalling tactic. Through this not-so-subtle form of obstructionism, we see the use of political hacks to fill governmental roles in the hope that nothing will happen. Think Hurricane Katrina, FEMA.

I met Danny twenty-three years ago. He was sitting on his mother's lap, a robust, full-cheeked six-month-old with the brownest, most knowing eyes I had ever seen in an infant. "There's something wrong," Sarina said. Her voice was strong, her gaze direct.

"Wrong?" I repeated. "He looks fine to me."

"That's what all the other doctors say, but I know different."

There was no denying Sarina, whose position in front of the doorway made it clear I was going to listen to her story. Danny had been born to a mother who showed up one day in the hospital, delivered, and left, never to be seen again. Sarina took Danny into her home three days after his birth; he has been living with her since. Experience with her own children and grandchildren gave Sarina the feeling right away that something was wrong. Danny was irritable and inconsolable. He pulled away from her when she tried to hold him close, and the more she consoled him the worse he got. There were two episodes when he seemed to "go blank," turning from her and staring at the opposite wall. His feeding was erratic, and although he would eventually drink the appropriate amount of formula, it took hours to feed him. It seemed that one feeding would run right into the next.

Sarina took Danny to a series of doctors, but the advice was always the same. "You're too old to be taking care of a new baby. Go home, relax, and call DCFS to come get him." Whether out of pity or pure stubbornness, Sarina ignored them all. She heard about our center from another foster mother, scheduled an immediate appointment, and appeared early one morning poised and ready for anyone who tried to turn her away.

During the examination, Danny lay quietly, giving way to tremors and irritability when I disturbed him. He had the physical signs of alcohol exposure. His eyes were set wide apart and his face appeared flattened. The bridge of the nose was flat and broad; his lips looked thin;

and his ears were situated low on the sides of his head, almost meeting the jaw line. Although well nourished, he was underweight; his length and head size fell far below normal for a six-month-old child. In the clinic, his behavior would escalate rapidly, reaching a peak of crying and shaking, before he would suddenly fall into a deep, impenetrable sleep.When the exam was finished, Sarina and I returned to the respective sides of the lone desk in the office. "Do you know anything about his mother?" I asked, watching her cuddle Danny in her arms as she tried to comfort him.

"No, that's all DCFS had," she said.

"Well, with nothing more to go on, I can't really say anything for sure. But Danny looks like a child whose mother used alcohol and drugs." Sarina nodded. Normally it's a hard sell to convey this information to a foster mother, but Sarina had made her own diagnosis, months ago. "I know," she said.

As she sat and listened, I outlined the various tests and procedures we would put Danny through over the next several days. She took in the information, patiently, in what I would learn was her usual style: gather the facts, ask questions, make a decision. Patty came into the room to draw blood, Eilene scheduled the necessary tests at the hospital, and Sarina agreed to return in one week to get the results.

The week went quickly until the day Danny's results came back from the hospital. He was HIV positive. I caught my breath, said a short prayer, and moved on.

Sarina appeared the next week, again wheedling for the first appointment in the morning, probably hoping to catch me at my freshest. "Sarina, the news isn't good." I was stumbling over my words as I tried to explain to her what the positive results meant to her son. "At this young age, we don't know if it's positive because he actually caught AIDS from his mother or it's positive because he was just exposed and not infected. There's about a 30%

chance he actually will have AIDS, but we won't know for sure until he's about fifteen months old." The last words came out in a rush. I realized I'd been holding my breath. Sarina sat quietly for a moment.

"What'll we do?" she asked. I told her we had to wait and see.

The next several months were spent in watchful anticipation. Danny continued to struggle with the normal developmental milestones that most infants breeze through. The arrhythmia of days filled with doctors and needles collapsed into restless nights punctuated by brief blessings of sleep. His adoption went through, and Sarina was on her own with no further support from DCFS.

By two years of age, an HIV test that remained positive and a series of illnesses confirmed Danny's diagnosis of AIDS. He and Sarina lived a life circumscribed by medication schedules, doctors' appointments, and feeding strategies to try to fatten him up. When Danny was three years old, a neighbor from the apartment building came to visit. Seeing a book on the coffee table, she commented, "Oh, now I know why Danny's sick all the time. He has AIDS." Sarina confirmed the neighbor's suspicions. A few days later, a petition, signed by almost all of the tenants in the building, requested that Sarina and her family vacate the building. The courts said, "No," and they remained in their home.

In eighth grade, Danny decided to go out for the middle school basketball team. His illness was a well-known fact by this time and had been handled quite well by the school district. It came as a surprise when the eighth grade mothers presented a petition to the coach stating that if Danny were allowed to play, they would not allow their sons to be on the team. The eighth grade boys responded in kind with their own petition: "If Danny doesn't play, we don't play." The children won out, and Danny became a member of the team. In a made-for-TV movie, Danny would have come off the bench and scored the winning points in the district championship game. But Danny was a pretty lousy player. Well meaning and a good sport, but clumsy with a basketball.

The next few years were spent in an unremitting cycle of relapse and recovery, with T-cell levels rising and falling on what seemed to be a whim. School was a struggle: reading and learning disabilities impeded Danny's comprehension of core elements of the basic curriculum.

During his freshman year, at the age of fifteen, he made an appointment with me. He arrived at my office with his fourteen-year-old girlfriend. They were going to have sex and wanted to know the best way to protect her. A fleeting surge of gratitude that they had come to discuss this with me quickly gave way to panic. I lectured, pleaded, and bargained with them—to no avail. So I sent them on their way with the best advice I could give. "Wear three rubbers." I knew this was unreasonable and counter to any scientific evidence, but I figured by the time he got the third rubber on, the desire would be gone. My strategy worked: three days later Danny called me to report that he and his girlfriend had broken up without consummating their relationship. I was ecstatic; Danny was heartbroken. I assured him that his time would come, just not yet.

All was relatively quiet for the next two years, but then Danny and Sarina appeared once again at my door. By this point Danny was on multiple medications, almost always sick from AIDS or the side effects of his prescriptions. At the age of seventeen, hardly able to go to school, he had made an end-of-life decision; he was stopping all his medications. We started with the facts as to what would happen if he stopped his meds. He understood the consequences. We resorted to begging. He was not swayed; he simply had had enough. Danny stopped his medications, and within two months he was hospitalized with seizures. The AIDS virus had invaded his brain. Miraculously, and for reasons not entirely clear, Danny was able to pull through. After a six-week course in the hospital he went home, scared enough by his experience to start the medications again. Then in 2003 a breakthrough came: Danny began taking a new, experimental AIDS cocktail.

Danny is now twenty-four years old and has no detectable AIDS virus. He calls me once a year on my birthday, and I get the occasional call from Sarina, whose main complaint is that Danny refuses to get a full time job because his band takes up all his energy and attention. He's quite sure that one day he'll make it to *American Idol*. Like his mother, Sarina, he isn't quick to sell himself short.

Addressing the GoodEnough Syndrome

We are a nation that professes to value children: *Primus inter parus* . . . Children are first among equals. However, when issues are put to balance other interests and investments take precedence. There is no point railing against those things we cannot change. In the arena of child welfare, extreme recommendations too often substitute for viable policy. Instead, here are a few simple and cost-effective policies we can pursue immediately to change the lives of children for the better.

- **Public health**

  Implement universal screening programs for all pregnant women that will identify those women at risk for alcohol, tobacco and illicit drug use, depression, or domestic violence. The purpose of such screening is to engage each woman in an educational intervention that will motivate her to make healthy decisions for herself and her unborn child; the purpose is not to make prenatal clinics an arm of the child welfare system.

- **Child welfare**

  Develop research-based policies for decision making regarding placement of children identified as at risk from prenatal alcohol or drug exposure. Within the CAPTA legislation, include prenatal alcohol exposure as a risk factor and create national guidelines that describe what it means to be an "affected" infant. Develop support systems and education and training programs for foster and adoptive parents who bring substance-exposed infants and children into their homes, so as to reduce the high rates of placement disruptions for the child.

- **Early intervention and treatment**

  Define service access to early intervention and treatment based on the child's needs rather than eligibility criteria. Eliminate the need for young children to meet *DSM-IV* criteria in order to qualify for mental health services. Rather, develop a nationally accepted "crosswalk" between functional diagnoses, such as those described in the *DC: 0-3* diagnostic scheme, and qualifying *DSM-IV* diagnoses. Expand early intervention services to include infant mental health programs.

We are caught downstream, trying to adapt families and children to existing policies and practices rather than promoting innovative approaches that address the new morbidity that exists among families and children in the United States. In so many ways, our children are drowning. Yet we continue to pour resources into rescuing our children from the river rather than traveling upstream to find out who's pushing them in. And why? Because it's easier to hide behind labels of risk than to work to improve children's lives.

In every way, Danny was — and is — a child "at risk." But Danny has a mother who shortcut the systems that blocked her access, ignored those professionals who told her all hope was lost, and refused to accept health, mental health, and educational systems that were *good enough* for a child with AIDS. Sarina accepted possibility but denied probability when "risk" was used to describe her child. She built on Danny's promise. And Danny not only survived, he flourished. The balance between risk and promise? That's the mystery of risk.

APPENDIX Policy Recommendations

The extraordinary efforts of clinicians and researchers across the country have borne fruit as we look at the progress being made in the field of perinatal addictions and child health and welfare. But present efforts are focused on only one aspect of the problem or another, and we continue to operate within the silos of our particular interests. The current situation provides an opportunity for leadership at both the federal and state level. Several approaches that have been implemented at one level or another in different parts of the country can serve as models for more successful overarching policies and procedures, especially at the state level. Although most states have no official statewide body that addresses the full range of effects of prenatal substance exposure on pregnancy and child outcome, such an organizational unit could be an important unifying focal point for action at the state level:

I. **Support defining and tracking the problem of substance use in pregnancy**
   1. Form a council of state and local agencies affected by the problem of prenatal substance exposure and develop baseline data from a variety of agency perspectives.
      a. Key agencies include Departments of Public Health, Health Care Services, Social Services (child welfare), Developmental Services (developmental disabilities), Alcohol and Drug Programs, Education, and Mental Health, to name a few.

    b. Present an annual state report compiled from county or other local jurisdictional submissions of data on prenatal screening and determine the feasibility of follow-up monitoring of birth results in relation to prenatal screening data.

2. Develop a centralized database and conduct periodic data compilation to track rates of positive screens for substance use in pregnant women. Louisiana and New Jersey track all perinatal substance use data acrossthe state, and Indiana conducts double-blind meconium screenings at birth as a baseline for prevalence.

3. Develop guidelines to support local and state Fetal/Infant Mortality Review committees in their efforts to assess, link, and track perinatal substance use and its impact on fetal and infant deaths and illnesses.

4. Redesign the federally mandated reporting systems for child welfare and substance abuse treatment to include information about substance use disorders affecting child welfare cases, pregnancy status, and admission to treatment of prenatally screened clients.

II. Support prevention, identification, and intervention efforts

1. Develop and implement local and statewide prevention campaigns to address substance use in pregnancy.

    a. Focus separate messages on the particular populations documented to be at highest risk for using alcohol, tobacco, and illicit drugs in early pregnancy and continuing that use through pregnancy.

    b. Provide prevention materials for clinicians in primary prenatal care and associated settings to support individual prevention/intervention approaches during preconception and pregnancy.

    c. Link new steps to existing efforts regarding prevention of tobacco use.

2. Support studies of substance use in pregnant women across the array of racial and ethnic identities in each state.
   a. Identify unique risk factors and patterns of use within each population of women.
   b. Define intervention points across the social and health care spectrum.
   c. Develop culturally appropriate community education and prevention campaigns.
3. Make screening for substance use, depression, and domestic violence in a family part of routine prenatal care.
   a. Encourage use of validated questions for substance use screening among all providers.
   b. Avoid invasive strategies such as using urine toxicologies to screen for substance use.
   c. Support existing efforts to make screening and intervention fully reimbursable by Medicaid and private insurance providers, utilizing appropriate billing codes to take advantage of new federal Medicaid regulations that allow payment for screening and brief intervention in the primary care setting.
   d. Work with private insurers to develop support for screening and brief intervention in the primary prenatal care setting.
4. Review current hospital practice and compliance with federal Child Abuse Prevention and Treatment Act (CAPTA) legislation.
   a. Educate physicians and other hospital personnel as to their responsibilities for identifying and reporting newborns affected by prenatal substance exposure.
   b. Ensure child welfare workers investigating such cases are fully aware of the risks for the newborns and the variety of appropriate interventions available for mothers and infants.

    c. Strengthen the link between child welfare and early infant intervention services in each state, ensuring that all children at risk have the benefit of early intervention services.

    d. Discourage any attempts to criminalize a mother's giving birth to a prenatally exposed infant. Promote dyadic treatment approaches that support the woman's recovery and the child's ultimate welfare.

5. Ensure all children have access to appropriate intervention and treatment services.

    a. Expand eligibility criteria for early intervention and special education services in all states to include children at risk from prenatal exposure to alcohol or illicit drugs.

    b. Require Part C early intervention agencies to report annually on CAPTA referrals they receive from child protection services agencies and their disposition of these referrals.

    c. Utilize "functional diagnoses," as derived from the *DC: 0-3* diagnostic system, to determine clinician's reimbursement for caring for young children with mental health disorders. Terminate reliance on *DSM* criteria for diagnosis and, hence, treatment eligibility of young children birth to five years of age.

6. Raise alcohol excise taxes in every state. This is a proven strategy for reducing excessive drinking and its associated harm and could provide a source of revenue for FAS prevention efforts.

7. In each county, in every state, promote the development of an integrated system of care that spans a continuum. This includes preconception prevention messages and support for both children and parents affected by perinatal substance exposure, including substance use prevention and family planning services for women.

8. Produce guidelines for offering pregnancy testing and contraceptive services to all women entering substance abuse treatment and for linking pregnant women in substance abuse treatment programs to prenatal care.

9. Develop and provide cross-training programs for staff working in agencies and programs that have access to pregnant women and their children:
   a. Prenatal care providers
   b. Pediatricians and other child health care providers
   c. Substance abuse treatment providers
   d. Child welfare professionals
   e. Educators
   f. Judges and other court personnel

III. Build and sustain support for integrated systems of care for pregnant women and their children affected by prenatal substance use

10. Develop relationships with and obtain endorsement from local and statewide associations of medical personnel to support universal screening of pregnant women

11. Determine and assess the perinatal substance use efforts implemented by existing agencies and programs in each state and the resulting best practice models for perinatal substance use screening and identification of children at risk from prenatal exposure.

There are those who would protest that these policies would impose too great a financial burden on federal, state, and local governments. However, we already are bearing this burden at two to three times greater cost due to our preference for rescuing children rather than preventing and directly addressing these tragedies.

Bibliography

ADOLESCENCE

Cicchetti D, Rogosch FA. A developmental psychopathology perspective on adolescence. *Journal of Consulting and Clinical Psychology.* 2002;70(1):6–20.

Duquette C, Stodel E, Fullarton S, Haggulnd K. Persistence in high school: experiences of adolescents and young adults with fetal alcohol spectrum disorder. *Journal of Intellectual and Developmental Disability.* 2006;31(4):219–231.

Hooper CJ, Luciana M, Conklin HM, Yarger RS. Adolescents' performance on the development of decision making and ventromedial prefrontal cortex. *Developmental Psychology.* 2004;40:1148–1158.

Luciana M, Conklin HM, Cooper CJ, Yarger RS. The development of nonverbal working memory and executive control processes in adolescents. *Child Development.* 2005;76:697–712.

Resnick MD, Bearman PS, Blum RW, Bauman KE, Harris KM, Jones J. Protecting adolescents from harm. Findings from the National Longitudinal Study on Adolescent Health. *Journal of the American Medical Association.* 1997;278:823–832.

Shaw P, Greenstein D, Lerch J, et al. (2006). Intellectual ability and cortical development in children and adolescents. *Nature.* 2006;440, 676–679.

Spohr, H. Fetal alcohol syndrome in adolescence: long-term perspective of children diagnosed in infancy. In: Spohr H, Steinhausen H, eds. *Alcohol, Pregnancy, and the Developing Child.* New York, NY: Cambridge University Press; 1996:207–226.

ATTACHMENT AND PARENT-CHILD RELATIONSHIPS

Butterfield P, Martin C, Praire A. *Emotional Connections: How Relationships Guide Early Learning.* Washington, DC: Zero to Three Press; 2004.

Clark R, Tluczek A, Gallagher KC. Assessment of parent-child early relational disturbances. In: DelCarmen-Wiggins R, Carter A, eds. *Handbook of Infant, Toddler, and Pre-school Mental Health Assessment.* New York, NY: Oxford University Press; 2004.

Dunn, W. A sensory processing approach to supporting infant-caregiver relationships. In: Sameroff A, McDonough S, Rosenblum K, eds. *Treating Parent-Infant Relationship Problems.* New York, NY: The Guildford Press; 2004:152–187.

Farina L, Leifer M, Chasnoff IJ. Attachment and behavioural difficulties in internationally adopted Russian orphans. *Adoption and Fostering*. 2004;28:38–48.

Fox N, Polak C. The role of sensory reactivity in understanding infant temperament. In: DesCarmen R, Carter A, eds. *Handbook of Infant, Toddler, and Preschool Mental Health Assessment*. New York, NY: Oxford University Press; 2004: 105–122.

Glaser D. Child abuse and neglect and the brain – a review. *Journal of Child Psychology and Psychiatry*. 2000;41:97–116.

Goleman, D. *Social Intelligence: The New Science of Human Relationships*. New York, NY: Bantam Books; 2006.

Greenspan S, Porges S. Psychopathology in infancy and early childhood: clinical perspectives on the organization of sensory and affective-thematic experience. *Child Development*. 1984;55(1):49–70.

Greenspan S, Wieder S. *Engaging Autism: Using the Floortime Approach to Help Children Relate, Communicate and Think*. Cambridge, MA: DaCapo Press; 2006a.

Greenspan S, Wieder S. *Infant and Early Childhood Mental Health: A Comprehensive Developmental Approach to Assessment and Intervention*. Washington, DC: American Psychiatric Publishing, Inc; 2006b.

Kaye K. *The Mental and Social Life of Babies: How Parents Create Persons*. Chicago: University of Chicago Press; 1982.

Porges S. Neuroception: A subconscious system for detecting threats and safety. *Zero To Three*. 2004;19-24.

Schore AN. Attachment and the regulation of the right brain. *Attachment and Human Development*. 2000;2:23–47.

Schore AN. *Affect Regulation and the Origin of the Self: The Neurobiology of Emotional Development*. Hillsdale, NJ: Lawrence Erlbaum Associates; 1994.

Siegel DJ. *The Developing Mind: How Relationships and the Brain Interact to Shape Who We Are*. New York, NY: The Guilford Press; 1999.

Smyke A, Dumitrescu A, Zeanah C. Attachment disturbances in young children: the continuum of caretaking casualty. *Journal of the American Academy of Child and Adolescent Psychiatry*. 2002;41(8):972–982.

Sroufe L. Emotional Development: *The Organization of Emotional Life in the Early Years*. New York, NY: The Cambridge University Press; 1995.

Stifter C, Wiggins C. Assessment of disturbances in emotional regulation and temperament. In: DesCarmen R, Carter A, eds. *Handbook of Infant, Toddler, and Preschool Mental Health Assessment*. New York, NY: Oxford University Press; 2004: 79–194.

Tronick E. *The Neurobehavioral and Social-Emotional Development of Infants and Young Children*. New York, NY: W.W. Norton and Co; 2007.

ATTENTION-DEFICIT / HYPERACTIVITY DISORDER
Barkley RA. *Attention-Deficit Hyperactivity Disorder: A Handbook for Diagnosis and Treatment*. 2nd ed. New York, NY: Guilford Press; 1998.

Brookes KJ, Mill J, Guindalini C, et al. A common haplotype of the dopamine transporter gene associated with attention-deficit/hyperactivity disorder and interacting with maternal use of alcohol during pregnancy. *Archives of General Psychiatry*. 2006;63(1):74–81.

Jensen PS. ADHD: Current concepts on etiology, pathophysiology, and neurobiology. *Child and Adolescent Psychiatric Clinics of North America*. 2000;9:557–572.

Lee KR, Mattson SN, Riley EP. Classifying children with heavy prenatal alcohol exposure using measures of attention. *Journal of the International Neuropsychological Society*. 2004;10:271–277.

Mattson SN, Calarco KE, Lang AR. Focused and shifting attention in children with heavy prenatal alcohol exposure. *Neuropsychology*. 2006;20:361–369.

Palfrey JS, Levine MD, Walker DK, et al. The emergence of attention deficits in early childhood: A prospective study. *Journal of Developmental and Behavioral Pediatrics*. 1985;6:339–348.

Pliszka SR, McCracken, JT, Maas JW. Catecholamines in attention-deficit hyperactivity disorder: current perspectives. *Journal of the American Academy of Child and Adolescent Psychiatry*. 1996;35:264–272.

Swanson J, Castellanos FX, Murias M, et al: Cognitive neuroscience of attention deficit hyperactivity disorder and hyperkinetic disorder. *Current Opinion in Neurobiology*. 1998;8:263–271.

Zametkin AJ, Rapoport JL. Neurobiology of attention deficit disorder with hyperactivity: Where have we come in 50 years? *Journal of the American Academy of Child and Adolescent Psychiatry*. 1987;26:676–686.

ECONOMICS OF FETAL ALCOHOL SPECTRUM DISORDERS

Abel, EL, Sokol, RJ. A revised conservative estimate of the incidence of FAS and its economic impact. *Alcoholism: Clinical and Experimental Research*. 1991;15(3):514.

Abel EL and Sokol RJ. Incidence of Fetal Alcohol Syndrome and economic impact of FAS-related anomalies. *Drug and Alcohol Dependence*. 1987;19:51–70.

Harwood HJ, Napolitano DM. Economic implications of the Fetal Alcohol syndrome. *Alcohol Health and Research World*. 1985;Fall:38–43.

EXECUTIVE FUNCTIONING

Barkley RA. The executive functions and self-regulation: an evolutionary neuropsychological perspective. *Neruopsychology Review*. 2001;11:1–29.

Coles CD, Platzman KA, Raskind-Hood CL, Brown RT, Falek A, Smith IE. A comparison of children affected by prenatal alcohol exposure and attention deficit hyperactivity disorder. *Alcoholism: Clinical & Experimental Research*. 1997;26:263–271.

Connor PD, Sampson PD, Bookstein FL, Barr HM, Streissguth AP. Direct and indirect effects of prenatal alcohol damage on executive function. *Developmental Neuropsychology*. 2000;18:331–354.

Fryer SL, Tapert SF, Mattson SN, Paulus MP, Spadoni AD, Riley EP. Prenatal alcohol exposure affects frontal-striatal response during inhibitory control. *Alcoholism: Clinical and Experimental Research.* 2007;31(8):1415-1424.

Hanna-Pladdy, B. Dysexecutive syndromes in neurologic disease. *Journal of Neurologic Physical Therapy.* 2007;31:119-127.

Kodituwakku PW, May PA, Clericuzio CL, Weers D. Emotion-related learning in individuals prenatally exposed to alcohol: An investigation of the relation between set shifting, extinction of responses, and behavior. *Neuropsychologia.* 2001;39:699-708.

Mattson SN, Goodman AM, Caine C, Delis DC, Riley EP. Executive functioning in children with heavy prenatal alcohol exposure. *Alcoholism: Clinical and Experimental Research.* 1999;23:1808-1815.

Mayes LC. A developmental perspective on the regulation of arousal states. *Seminars in Perinatology.* 2000;24:267-279.

Noland JS, Singer LT, Arendt RE, Minnes S, Short EJ, Bearer CF. Executive functioning in preschool-age children prenatally exposed to alcohol, cocaine, and marijuana. *Alcoholism: Clinical and Experimental Research.* 2003;27:647-656.

Schonfeld AM, Mattson SN, Lang AR, Delis DC, Riley EP. Verbal and nonverbal fluency in children with heavy prenatal alcohol exposure. *Journal of Studies on Alcohol.* 2001;62:239-246.

FETAL ALCOHOL SYNDROME

Astley SJ. Comparison of the 4-digit diagnostic code and the Hoyme diagnostic guidelines for Fetal Alcohol Spectrum Disorders. *Pediatrics.* 2006;118:1532-1545.

Astley SJ, Aylward EH, Olson HC, et al. Magnetic resonance imaging outcomes from a comprehensive magnetic resonance study of children with fetal alcohol spectrum disorders. *Alcoholism: Clinical and Experimental Research.* 2009;33:1671-1689.

Astley SJ, Clarren SK. Diagnosing the full spectrum of fetal alcohol-exposed individuals: introducing the 4-digit diagnostic code. *Alcohol & Alcoholism.* 2000;35:400-412.

Astley SJ, Olson HC, Kerns K, et al. Neuropsychological and behavioral outcomes from a comprehensive magnetic resonance study of children with fetal alcohol spectrum disorders. *Canadian Journal of Clinical Pharmacology.* 2009;16:e178-e201.

Bertrand J, Floyd L, Chasnoff IJ, Wells A, Bailey G, et al. Interventions for children with fetal alcohol spectrum disorders (FASD): Overview of findings for five innovative research projects. *Research in Developmental Disabilities.* 2009;986-1006.

Bertrand J, Floyd RL, Weber MK. Guidelines for identifying and referring persons with fetal alcohol syndrome. *Morbidity and Mortality Weekly Report.* 2005;54:1-15.

Bertrand J, Floyd RL, Weber MK, et al. National Task Force on FAS/FAE. Fetal Alcohol Syndrome: Guidelines for Referral and Diagnosis; 2004; Atlanta, GA: Centers for Disease Control and Prevention.

Carmichael Olson, H, Feldman JJ, Streissguth AP, Sampson PD, Bookstein FL. Neuropsychological deficits in adolescents with Fetal Alcohol Syndrome: clinical findings. *Alcoholism: Clinical & Experimental Research.* 1998;22(9):1998–2012

Carmichael Olson H, Streissguth AP, Sampson, PD, Barr HM, Bookstein, FL, Thiede, K. Association of prenatal alcohol exposure with behavioral and learning problems in early adolescence. *Journal of the American Academy of Child and Adolescent Psychiatry.* 1997;36(9):1187–1194.

Chasnoff IJ. *The Nature of Nurture: Behavior, Environment, and the Drug-Exposed Child.* Chicago, IL: NTI Publishing; 2002.

Chasnoff IJ, McGourty RF, Bailey GF, et al. *The 4P's Plus*© Screen for substance use in pregnancy: Clinical application and outcomes. *Journal of Perinatology.* 2005;25:368-374.

Chasnoff IJ, Wells AM, Telford E, Schmidt C, Messer G. Neurodevelopmental functioning in children with FAS, pFAS, and ARND. *Journal of Developmental and Behavioral Pediatrics.* 2010; in press.

Clark CM, Li DC, Conry J, Loock R. Structural and functional brain integrity of Fetal Alcohol Syndrome in Nonretarded Cases. *Pediatrics.* 2000;105:1096 ISSN 0031-4005.

Coles CD, Brown RT, Smith IE, Platzman KA, Erickson S, Falek A. Effects of prenatal alcohol exposure at school age: I. Physical and cognitive development. *Neurotoxicology and Teratology.* 1991;13:357–367.

Coles C, Platzman K, Raskind-Hood C, Brown R, Falek A, Smith I. A comparison of children affected by prenatal alcohol exposure and attention deficit hyperactivity disorder. *Alcoholism: Clinical and Experimental Research.* 1997;21(1):150–161.

Day NL, Leech SL, Richardson GA, et al. Prenatal alcohol exposure predicts continued deficits in offspring size at 14 years of age. *Alcoholism: Clinical and Experimental Research.* 2002;26(10):1584–1591.

Day NL, Robies N, Richardson G, et al. The Effects of Prenatal Alcohol Use on the Growth of Children at Three Years of Age. *Alcoholism: Clinical and Experimental Research.* 1991;15(1):67–71.

Disney ER, Iacono W, McGue M, Tully E, Legrand L. Strengthening the case: prenatal alcohol exposure is associated with increased risk for conduct disorder. Pediatrics. 2008;122; e1225–e1230. doi:10.1542/peds.2008-1380.

D'Onofio BM, Van Hulle CA, Waldman ID, Rodgers JL, Rathouz PJ, Lahey BB. Causal inferences regarding prenatal alcohol exposure and childhood externalizing problems. *Archives of General Psychiatry.* 2007;64(11):1296–1304.

Fryer SL, McGee CL., Matt GE, Riley EP, Mattson SN. Evaluation of psychopathological conditions in children with heavy prenatal alcohol exposure. *Pediatrics.* 2007;119(3). Available at: www.pediatrics.org/cgi/content/full/119/3/e733.

Howell KK, Lynch ME, Platzman KA, Smith GH, Coles CD. Prenatal alcohol exposure and ability, academic achievement, and school functioning in adolescence: a longitudinal follow-up. *Journal of Pediatric Psychology.* 2006;31(1):116–126.

Hoyme HE, May PA, Kalberg WO, et al. A practical clinical approach to diagnosis of Fetal Alcohol Spectrum Disorders: Clarificaton of the 1996 Institute of Medicine Criteria. *Pediatrics.* 2005;115:39–47.

Jacobson S, Jacobson J, Sokol RJ, Martier S. and Ager J. Prenatal alcohol exposure and infant information processing ability. *Child Development.* 1993;64:1706–1721.

Jones K, Smith DW. Recognition of the fetal alcohol syndrome in early infancy. *Lancet.* 1973;ii:999–1201.

Kaemingk KL, Mulvaney S, Tanner Halverson P. Learning following prenatal alcohol exposure: performance on verbal and visual multi-trial tasks. *Archives of Clinical Neuropsychology.* 1993;18:33–47.

Kerns K, Don A, Mateer C, Striessguth AP. Cognitive deficits in nonretarded adults with fetal alcohol syndrome. *Journal of Learning Disabilities.* 1997;30(6):685–693.

Kesmodel, U, et al. Moderate alcohol intake during pregnancy and the risk of stillbirth and death in the first year of life. *American Journal of Epidemiology.* February 15, 2002(4)155(4):305–312.

Knopik VS, Health AC, Jacob T, et al. Maternal alcohol use disorder and offspring ADHD: disentangling genetic and environmental effects using a children-of-twins design. *Psychological Medicine.* 2006;36(10):1461–1471.

Kodituwakku, P.W. Defining the behavioral phenotype in children with fetal alcohol spectrum disorders: A review. *Neuroscience and Biobehavioral Reviews.* 2007;31:192–201.

Larroque B, Kaminski M. Prenatal alcohol exposure and development at preschool: Main results of a French study. *Alcoholism: Clinical and Experimental Research.* 1998;22(2):295–303.

Larroque B, Kaminski M, Dehaene P, Subtil D, Querleu D. Prenatal alcohol exposure and signs of minor neurological dysfunction at preschool-age. *Developmental Medicine and Child Neurology.* 2000;42:508–514.

Lemoine P, Harousseau H, Borteyru JP, Nenuet JC. Les enfants des parents alcoholiques: Anomlies observees a propos de 127 cas [The children of alcoholic parents: anomalies observed in 127 cases]. *Ouest Medical.* 1968;8:476–482.

Mattson SN, Calarco KE, Lang AR. Focused and shifting attention in children with heavy prenatal alcohol exposure. *Neuropsychology.* 2006;20(3):361–369.

Mattson SN, Jernigan TL, Riley EP. MRI and prenatal alcohol exposure. *Alcohol Health & Research World.* 1994;18:49–52.

Mattson SN, Riley EP. Prenatal exposure to alcohol: What the images reveal. *Alcohol Health & Research World.* 1995;19:273–277.

Mattson SN, Riley EP, Gramling L, Dellis DC, Jones KL. Heavy prenatal alcohol exposure with or without physical features of Fetal Alcohol Syndrome leads to IQ deficits. *Journal of Pediatrics.* 1997;131:718–721.

Mattson SN, Riley EP, Gramling L, Delis DC, Jones KL. Neuropsychological comparison of alcohol-exposed children with or without physical features of Fetal Alcohol Syndrome. *Neuropsychology.* 1998;12:46–153.

Mattson SN, Riley EP, Sowell ER, Jernigan TL, Sobel DF, Jones KL. A decrease in the size of the basal ganglia in children with fetal alcohol syndrome. *Alcoholism: Clinical and Experimental Research.* 1996;20:1088–1093.

Nanson JL, Hiscock M. Attention deficits in children exposed to alcohol prenatally. *Alcoholism: Clinical and Experimental Research.* 1990;14:656–661.

O'Callaghan FV, O'Callaghan M. Najman JM, Najman JM, Williams GM, Bor. W. Prenatal alcohol exposure and attention, learning and intellectual ability at 14 years: a prospective longitudinal study. *Early Human Development.* 2007;83(2):115–123.

Rasmussen C, Horne K, Witol A. Neurobehavioral functioning in children with Fetal Alcohol Spectrum Disorder. *Child Neuropsychology.* 2006;12:1–16.

Richardson GA, Ryan C. Willford J. Day NL, Goldschmidt L. Prenatal alcohol and marijuana exposure: effects on neuropsychological outcomes at 10 years. *Neurotoxicology and Teratology.* 2002;24:309–320.

Riley EP, McGee CL. Fetal Alcohol Spectrum Disorders: An overview with emphasis on changes in brain and behavior. *Experimental Biology and Medicine.* 2005;230:357–365.

Roebuck TM, Mattson SN, Riley EP. A review of the neuroanatomical findings in children with FAS. *Clinical and Experimental Research.* 1998;22:339–344.

Roebuck-Spencer TM, Mattson SN. Implicit strategy affects learning in children with heavy prenatal alcohol exposure. *Alcoholism: Clinical and Experimental Research.* 2004;28:1424–1431.

Sampson PD, Streissguth AP, Bookstein FL, et al. Incidence of Fetal Alcohol Syndrome and prevalence of alcohol-related neurodevelopmental disorder. *Teratology.* 1997;56:317–326.

Sayal K. Alcohol consumption in pregnancy as a risk factor for later mental health problems. *Evidence-Based Mental Health.* 2007;10(4):98–100.

Schonfeld AM, Mattson SN, Lang AR, Delis DC, Riley EP. Verbal and nonverbal fluency in children with heavy prenatal alcohol exposure. *Journal of Studies on Alcohol.* 2001;62, 239–246.

Schonfeld AM, Mattson SN, Riley EP. Moral maturity and delinquency after prenatal alcohol exposure. *Journal of Studies on Alcohol.* 2005;66:545–554.

Sokol, RJ, et al. Fetal Alcohol Spectrum Disorder. *Journal of the American Medical Association.* 2003;290(22): 2996–2999.

Sood, B, et al. Prenatal Alcohol Exposure and Childhood Behavior at Age 6 to 7. *Pediatrics.* 2001;108(2):e34.

Steinhausen H, Willms J, Spohr H. Long-term psychopathological and cognitive outcome of children with fetal alcohol syndrome. *Journal of the American Academy of Child and Adolescent Psychiatry.* 1993;32(5):990–995.

Stratton K, Howe C, Battaglia F, eds. *Fetal Alcohol Syndrome: Diagnosis, Epidemiology, Prevention, and Treatment.* Washington, DC: National Academy Press, Institute of Medicine; 1996.

Streissguth A. Offspring effects of prenatal alcohol exposure from birth to 25 years: The Seattle prospective longitudinal study. *Journal of Clinical Psychology in Medical Settings.* 2007;14:81–101.

Streissguth, A. *Fetal Alcohol Syndrome: A Guide for Families and Communities.* Baltimore, MD: Paul H. Brooks Publishing Co; 1997.

Streissguth A, Bookstein F, Sampson P, Barr H. *The Enduring Effects of Prenatal Alcohol Exposure on Child Development: Birth Through Seven Years, a Partial Least Squares Solution.* Ann Arbor, MI: The University of Michigan Press; 1993.

Streissguth A, Kanter J. *The Challenge of Fetal Alcohol Syndrome: Overcoming Secondary Disabilities.* Seattle, WA: University of Washington Press; 1997.

Streissguth AP, Aase JM, Clarren SK, Randels SP, LaDue RA, Smith DF. Fetal Alcohol Syndrome in adolescents and adults. *The Journal of the American Medical Association.* 1991;265:1961–1967.

Streissguth, AP, et al. Risk factors for adverse life outcomes in Fetal Alcohol Syndrome and Fetal Alcohol Effects. *Journal of Developmental and Behavioral Pediatrics.* 2004;25(4):228–238.

Suess P, Newlin D, Porges S. Motivation, sustained attention, and autonomic regulation in school-age boys exposed in utero to opiates and alcohol. *Experimental and Clinical Psychopharmacology.* 1997;5(4):375–387.

Swayze VW, Johnson VP, Hanson JW, et al. Magnetic resonance imaging of brain anomalies in Fetal Alcohol Syndrome. *Pediatrics.* 1997;99:232–241.

Willford J, Leech S, Day N. Moderate prenatal alcohol exposure and cognitive status of children at age 10. *Alcoholism: Clinical and Experimental Research.* 2006;30(6):1051–1059.

FETAL DEVELOPMENT

Hepper PG. Adaptive fetal learning: prenatal exposure to garlic affects postnatal preference. *Animal Behavior.* 1988;36:935–936.

Hepper PG. Fetal memory: Does it exist? What does it do? *Acta Paediatrica.* 1996;Suppl 416:16-20. Stockholm. ISSN 0803-5326.

Hepper PG, Scott D, Shahdullah S. Newborn and fetal response to maternal voice. *Journal of Reproductive and Infant Psychology.* 1993;11:147–153.

Hepper PG, Shahdullah S. Development of fetal hearing. *Archives of Disease in Childhood.* 1994;71:F81–F87.

Lickliter R, Stoumbos J. Modification of prenatal auditory experience alters postnatal auditory preferences of bobwhite quail chicks. *The Quarterly Journal of Experimental Psychology.* 1992;44B:199–214.

Mennella JA, Beauchamp GK. Maternal diet alters the sensory qualities of human milk and the nursling's behavior. *Pediatrics.* 1991;88:737–744.

Moon C, Cooper RP, Fifer WP. Two-day-olds prefer their native language. *Infant Behavior & Development.* 1991;16:495–500.

Porter RH. Mutual mother-infant recognition in humans. In: Hepper PG ed. *Kin Recognition*. Cambridge, England: Cambridge University Press; 1991.

Querleu D, Renard X, Versyp F, Paris-Delrue L, Crepin G. Fetal hearing. *European Journal of Obstetrics & Gynecology and Reproductive Biology*. 1988;29:191-212.

Wilkin PE. Prenatal and postnatal responses to music and sound stimuli. In: Blum T ed. *Prenatal Perception Learning and Bonding*. Berlin: Leonardo; 1993.

ILLICIT DRUGS AND TOBACCO

Accornero VH, Amado AJ, Morrow CE, Xue L, Anthony JC, Bandstra ES. Impact of prenatal cocaine exposure on attention and response inhibition as assessed by continuous performance tests. *Journal of Developmental and Behavioral Pediatrics*. 2007;28(3):195-205.

Accornero VH, Anthony JC, Morrow CE, Xue L. Bandstra ES. Prenatal cocaine exposure: an examination of childhood externalizing and internalizing behavior problems at age 7 years. *Epidemiologia e Psichiatria Sociale*. 2006;15:20-29.

Ackerman JP, Llorente AM, Black MM, et al. The effect of prenatal drug exposure and caregiving context on children's performance on a task of sustained visual attention. *Journal of Developmental and Behavioral Pediatrics*. 2008;29;467-474.

Arendt RE, Short EJ, Singer LT, et al. Children prenatally exposed to cocaine: developmental outcomes and environmental risks at seven years of age. *Journal of Developmental and Behavioral Pediatrics*. 2004;25:83-90.

Azuma SD, Chasnoff IJ. Outcome of children prenatally exposed to cocaine and other drugs: A path analysis of three-year data. *Pediatrics*. 1993;92:396-402.

Bada HS, Das A, Bauer CR, et al. Low birth weight and preterm births: etiologic fraction attributable to prenatal drug exposure. *Journal of Perinatology*. 2005;25(10):631-637.

Bada HS, Das A, Bauer CR, et al. Impact of Prenatal Cocaine Exposure on Child Behavior Problems Through School Age. *Pediatrics* 2007;119:348-359 doi: 10.1542/peds.2006-1404.

Bailey BN, Hannigan JH, Delaney-Black V, Covington S, Sokol RJ. The role of maternal acceptance in the relation between community violence exposure and child functioning. *Journal of Abnormal Child Psychology*. 2006;34:57-70.

Bandstra ES, Morrow CE, Anthony JC, et al. Longitudinal investigation of task persistence and sustained attention in children with prenatal cocaine exposure. *Neurotoxicology and Teratology*. 2001;23:545-559.

Bauer RW. Methamphetamine in Illinois: an examination of an emerging drug. *Illinois Criminal Justice Information Authority Research Bulletin*. 2003;1(2):1-11.

Bauer CR, Langer JC, Shankaran S, et al. Acute neonatal effects of cocaine exposure during pregnancy. *Archives of Pediatrics & Adolescent Medicine*. 2005;159:824-834.

Beeghly M, Martin B, Rose-Jacobs R, et al. Prenatal cocaine exposure and children's language functioning at 6 and 9.5 years: moderating effects of child age, birth weight, and gender. *Journal of Pediatric Psychology*. 2006;31(1):98-115.

Behnke M, Eyler FD, Warner TD, Garvan CW, Hou W. Wobie K. Outcome from a prospective, longitudinal study of prenatal cocaine use: preschool development at 3 years of age. *Journal of Pediatric Psychology*. 2006;31:41–49.

Bennett D, Bendersky M, Lewis BA. Preadolescent health risk behavior as a function of prenatal cocaine exposure and gender. *Journal of Developmental and Behavioral Pediatrics*. 2007;28(6):467–472.

Cascio CJ, Gerig G, Piven J. Diffusion tensor imaging: application to the study of the developing brain. *Journal of the American Academy of Child and Adolescent Psychiatry*. 2007;46:213–223.

Chang L., Smith LM, LoPresti C, et al. Smaller subcortical volumes and cognitive deficits in children with prenatal methamphetamine exposure. *Psychiatry Research* 2004;132:95–106.

Chasnoff IJ. Effects of maternal narcotic vs. non-narcotic addiction on neonatal neurobehavior and infant development. In: Pinkert TM, ed. *Current Research on the Consequences of Maternal Drug Use*. Washington, DC: N.I.D.A.; 1985;59:84–95.

Chasnoff IJ. Drugs and alcohol in pregnancy and the affected child. In: Lessenger JE, Roper GF, eds. *Drug Courts: A New Approach to Treatment and Rehabilitation*. Springer Publishing; 2007.

Chasnoff IJ, Anson A, Hatcher R, Stenson H, Iaukea K, Randolph L. Prenatal exposure to cocaine and other drugs: Outcome at four to six years. In: Harvey JA, Kosofsky BE, eds. *Cocaine Effects On the Developing Brain*. New York, NY: Annals of the New York Academy of Science; 1998:314–328.

Chasnoff IJ, Burns WJ. The moro reaction: a scoring system for neonatal narcotic withdrawal. *Developmental Medicine and Child Neurology*. 1984;26:484–489.

Chasnoff IJ, Burns WJ, Hatcher R. Polydrug - and methadone - addicted newborns: a continuum of impairment? *Pediatrics*. 1982;70:210–212.

Chasnoff IJ, Burns WJ, Schnoll SH. Perinatal addiction: maternal narcotic vs. non-narcotic use during pregnancy and its effects on infant development. In: *Problems of Drug Dependence 1983*. N.I.D.A.; 1984;49:220–226.

Chasnoff IJ, Burns WJ, Schnoll SH, Burns KA. Cocaine use in pregnancy. *New England Journal of Medicine*. 1985;313:666–669.

Chasnoff IJ, Bussey M, Savich R, Stack CA. Perinatal cerebral infarction and maternal cocaine use. *Journal of Pediatrics*. 1986;108:456–459.

Chasnoff IJ, Griffith DR, MacGregor S, Dirkes K, Burns KA. Temporal patterns of cocaine use in pregnancy: perinatal outcome. *The Journal of the American Medical Association*. 1989;261(12):1741–1744.

Chasnoff IJ, Landress HJ, Barrett ME. The prevalence of illicit-drug or alcohol use during pregnancy and discrepancies in mandatory reporting in Pinellas County, Florida. *New England Journal of Medicine*. 1990;322:1202–1206.

Chasnoff IJ, Link JA. Environmental Tobacco Smoke: Office-Based Strategies for Prevention and Intervention. American Medical Association Secondhand Smoke Initiative Web site. http://www.ama-assn.org/ama/pub/physician-resources/

public-health/promoting-healthy-lifestyles/smoking-tobacco-control/ secondhand-smoke.shtml. Accessed Feb. 22, 2010.

Gendle MH, White TL, Strawderman M, et al. Enduring effects of prenatal cocaine exposure on selective attention and reactivity to errors: Evidence from an animal model. *Behavioral Neuroscience*. 2004;118:290–297.

Harris J. Drug-endangered children. *FBI Law Enforcement Bulletin*. February 2004;8–11.

Harvey JA. Cocaine effects on the developing brain: Current status. *Neuroscience and Biobehavioral Reviews*. 2004;27:751–764.

Hurt H, Brodsky NL, Roth H, Malmud E, Giannetta JM. School performance of children with gestational cocaine exposure. *Neurotoxicology and Teratology*. 2005;27(2):203–11.

Hurt H, Giannetta JM, Korczykowski M, et al. Functional magnetic resonance imaging and working memory in adolescents with gestational cocaine exposure. *Journal of Pediatrics*. 2008;152(3):371–377.

Kilbride HW, Castro CA, Fuger KL. School-age outcome of children with prenatal cocaine exposure following early case management. *Journal of Developmental and Behavioral Pediatrics*. 2006;27(3):181–187.

Lester BM, Tronick EZ, LaGasse L., et al. The maternal lifestyle study; effects of substance exposure during pregnancy on neurodevelopmental outcome in 1-month-old infants. *Pediatrics*. 2002;110:182–1192.

Linares TJ, Singer LT, Kirchner HL, et al. Mental health outcomes of cocaine-exposed children at 6 years of age. *Journal of Pediatric Psychology*. 2006;31:85–97.

Lumeng JC, Cabral HJ, Gannon K, Heeren T, Frank DA. Prenatal exposures to cocaine and alcohol and physical growth patterns to age 8 years. *Neurotoxicology and Teratology*. 2007;29(4)446–457.

Mayes LC. A behavioral teratogenic model of the impact of prenatal cocaine exposure on arousal regulatory systems. *Neurotoxicology and Teratology*. 2002;24:385–395.

Mayes LC, Molfese DL, Key AP, Hunter NC. Event-related potentials in cocaine-exposed children during a Stroop task. *Neurotoxicology and Teratology*. 2005;27:797–813.

McMahon J. What foster parents need to know about methamphetamine. *Fostering Perspectives*. 2005;9(2). http://www.fosterperspectives.org/fp_vol9no2/meth.htm.

Messinger DS, Bauer CR, Das A, et al. The maternal lifestyle study: cognitive, motor, and behavioral outcomes of cocaine-exposed and opiate-exposed infants through three years of age. *Pediatrics*. 2004;113;1677–1685.

Minnes S. Robin N, Alt A et al. Dysmorphic and anthropometric outcomes in 6-year-old prenatally cocaine-exposed children. *Neurotoxicology and Teratology*. 2006;28(1):28–38.

Morrow CE, Culbertson JL, Accornero VH, Xue L, Anthony JC, Bandstra ES. Learning disabilities and intellectual functioning in school-aged children with prenatal cocaine exposure. *Developmental Neuropsychology.* 2006;30:905–931.

Nair P, Black M, Ackerman J, Schuler M, Keane V. Children's cognitive-behavioral functioning at age 6 and 7: prenatal drug exposure and care giving environment. *Ambulatory Pediatrics.* 2008;8(3):154–162.

Noland JS, Singer LT, Arendt RE, Minnes S, Short EJ, Bearer CF. Executive functioning in preschool-age children prenatally exposed to alcohol, cocaine, and marijuana. *Alcoholism: Clinical and Experimental Research.* 2003;27(4):647–656.

Noland JS, Singer LT, Short EJ, Minnes S, Arendt RE, Kirchner HL, Bearer C. Prenatal drug exposure and selective attention in preschoolers. *Neurotoxicology and Teratology.* 2005;27:429–438.

Noland JS, Singer Ll, Short EJ, et al. Prenatal drug exposure and selective attention in preschoolers. *Neurotoxicology and Teratology.* 2005;27;429–438.

Nordstrom Bailey B, Sood BG, Sokol RJ, et al. Gender and alcohol moderate prenatal cocaine effects on teacher-report of child behavior. *Neurotoxicology and Teratology.* 2005;27(2):181–189.

Richardson GA, Goldschmidt L, Larkby C. Effects of prenatal cocaine exposure on growth: a longitudinal analysis. *Pediatrics.* 2007;120(4):e1017–1027.

Savage J, Brodsky NL, Malmud E, et al. Attentional functioning and impulse control in cocaine-exposed and control children at age ten years. *J Dev Beh Ped.* 2005;26:42–47.

Savage J, Brodsky NL, Malmud E. Giannetta JM, Hurt H. Attentional functioning and impulse control in cocaine-exposed and control children at age ten years. *Journal of Developmental and Behavioral Pediatrics.* 2005;26(1):42–47.

Schroder MD, Snyder PJ, Sielski I, Mayers L. Impaired performance of children exposed in utero to cocaine on a novel test of visuospatial working memory. *Brain and Cognition.* 2004;55:409–412.

Seifer R, LaGasse LL, Lester B, et al. Attachment status in children prenatally exposed to cocaine and other substances. *Child Development.* 2004;75:850–868.

Singer LT, Minnes S, Short E, et al. Cognitive outcomes of preschool children with prenatal cocaine exposure. *The Journal of the American Medical Association.* 2004;291:448–2456.

Singer LT, Nelson S, Short E, et al. Prenatal cocaine exposure: drug and environmental effects at 9 years. *Journal of Pediatrics.* 2008;153:105–111.

Smith LM, Lagasse LL., Derauf C, et al. Prenatal methamphetamine use and neonatal neurobehavioral outcome. *Neurotoxicology and Teratology.* 2008;30:20–28.

Smith L. Yonekura ML, Wallace T, Berman N, Kuo J, Berkowitz C. Effects of prenatal methamphetamine exposure on fetal growth and drug withdrawal symptoms in infants born at term. *J Dev Behav Pediatr.* 2003;24:17–23.

Warner TD, Behnke M, Eyler FD, et al. Diffusion tensor imaging of frontal white matter and executive functioning in cocaine-exposed children. *Pediatrics.* 2006;118:2014–2024.

Warner TD, Behnke M. Hous W. Garvan CW, Wobie K, Eyler FD. Predicting caregiver-reported behavior problems in cocaine-exposed children at 3 years. *Journal of Developmental and Behavioral Pediatrics.* 2006;27:83–92.

Webb RT, Wicks S, Dalman C, Pickles AR, Appleby L, Mortensen PB, Haglund B, Abel KM. Influence of environmental factors in higher risk of sudden infant death syndrome linked with parental mental illness. *Archives of General Psychiatry.* 2010;67:69–77.

Young NK. Children and Family Futures. Effects of methamphetamine on child welfare system. *Children and Family Futures.* May 31, 2006. http://wf2la6.webfeat. org/f9L1F1849/url=http://web.lexisnexis.com/unverse/printdoc.

MENTAL HEALTH

Barr HM, Bookstein FL, O'Malley KD, Connor PD, Huggins JF, Streissguth AP. Binge drinking during pregnancy as a predictor of psychiatric disorders on the Structured Clinical Interview for *DSM-IV* in young adult offspring. *American Journal of Psychiatry.* 2006;163:1061–1065.

Burns BJ, Phillips SD, Wagner HR, et al. J. Mental health need and access to mental health services by youth involved with child welfare: A national survey. *Journal of the American Academy of Child and Adolescent Psychiatry.* 2004;43:960–970.

Butterfield P, Martin C, Praire A. *Emotional Connections: How Relationships Guide Early Learning.* Washington, DC: Zero to Three Press; 2004.

Chasnoff IJ, Burns WJ, Schnoll SH, Burns K, Chisum G, Kyle-Spore L. Maternal/ Neonatal Incest. *American Journal of Orthopsychiatry.* 1986;56:577–580.

Famy C, Streissguth AP, Unis AS. Mental illness in adults with fetal alcohol syndrome or fetal alcohol effects. *American Journal of Psychiatry.* 1998;155:552–554.

Fryer SL, McGee CL, Matt GE, Riley EP. Evaluation of psychopathological conditions in children with heavy prenatal alcohol exposure. *Pediatrics.* 2007;119:733–741.

Lynch ME, Coles CD, Corley T, Falek A. Examining delinquency in adolescents differentially prenatally exposed to alcohol: The role of proximal and distal risk factors. *Journal of Studies on Alcohol.* 2003;64:678–686.

O'Connor MJ. Prenatal alcohol exposure and infant negative affect as precursors of depressive features in children. *Infant Mental Health Journal. Special Issue.* 2001;22:291–299.

O'Connor MJ, Kasari C. Prenatal alcohol exposure and depressive features in children. *Alcoholism: Clinical and Experimental Research.* 2000;24:1084–1092.

O'Connor MJ, Paley B. The relationship of prenatal alcohol exposure and the postnatal environment to child depressive symptoms. *Journal of Pediatric Psychology.* 2006;31:50–64.

O'Connor MJ, Shah B, Whaley S, Cronin P, Gunderson B, Graham J. Psychiatric illness in a clinical sample of children with prenatal alcohol exposure. *The American Journal of Drug and Alcohol Abuse.* 2002;28:743–754.

Shin SH. Need for and actual use of mental health service by adolescents in the child welfare system. *Children and Youth Services Review*. 2005;27:1071–1083.

Stifter C, Wiggins C.. Assessment of disturbances in emotional regulation and temperament. In: DesCarmen R, Carter A. *Handbook of Infant, Toddler, and Preschool Mental Health Assessment*. New York, NY: Oxford University Press; 2004.

Streissguth AP, Barr HM, Kogan J, Bookstein FL. *Understanding the Occurrence of Secondary Disabilities in Clients with Fetal Alcohol Syndrome (FAS) and Fetal Alcohol Effects (FAE): Final Report to The Centers for Disease Control and Prevention on Grant No. RO4/CCR008515*. Seattle, WA: University of Washington, Fetal Alcohol and Drug Unit; 1996. Tech Report No. 96-06.

Viner R, Taylor B. Adult health and social outcomes of children who have been in public care: Population-based study. *Pediatrics*. 2005;115:894–899.

PREVALENCE OF PRENATAL SUBSTANCE EXPOSURE
Abel EL, Sokol RJ. A revised conservative estimate of the incidence of FAS and its economic impact. *Alcoholism: Clinical and Experimental Research*. 1991;15:514–524.

Chasnoff IJ, Landress HJ, Barrett ME. The prevalence of drug or alcohol use during pregnancy and discrepancies in mandatory reporting in Pinellas County, Florida. *New England Journal of Medicine*. 1990;202–1206.

Chasnoff IJ, Wells AM, McGourty RF, McCurties S. *Perinatal Substance Use Screening in California: Screening and Assessment with the 4P's Plus© Screen for Substance Use in Pregnancy*. Sacramento, CA: California Department of Public Health: Maternal Child and Adolescent Health.; 2008.

Druschel CM, Fox DJ. Issues in estimating the prevalence of fetal alcohol syndrome: examination of 2 counties in New York state. *Pediatrics*. 2007;119;384–390. doi: 10.1542/peds.2006–0610.

May PA, Gossage JP, Kalberg WO, et al. Prevalence and epidemiologic characteristics of FASD from various research methods with an emphasis on recent in-school studies. *Developmental Disabilities Research Reviews*. 2009;15:176–192.

SENSORY INTEGRATION AND REGULATORY DISORDERS
Auer C, Blumberg S. *Parenting a Child with Sensory Processing Disorder: A Family Guide to Understanding and Supporting Your Sensory-Sensitive Child*. Oakland, CA: New Harbinger Publications; 2006.

Ben-Sasson A, Cermack S, Orsmond G, Carter A, Fogg L. Can we differentiate sensory over-responsivity form anxiety symptoms in toddlers? Perspectives of occupational therapists and psychologists. *Infant Mental Health Journal*. 2007;28(5): 536–558.

DeGangi G. *Pediatric Disorders of Regulation in Affect and Behavior: A Therapist's Guide to Assessment and Treatment*. San Diego, CA: Academic Press; 2000.

Dunn W. A sensory processing approach to supporting infant-caregiver relationships. In: Sameroff A, McDonough S, Rosenblum K, eds. *Treating Parent-Infant Relationship Problems*. New York, NY: The Guildford Press; 2004:152–187.

Fox N, Polak C. The role of sensory reactivity in understanding infant temperament. In: DesCarmen R, Carter A. *Handbook of Infant, Toddler, and Preschool Mental Health Assessment*. New York, NY: Oxford University Press; 2004:105–122.

Franklin L, Deitz J, Jirikowic T, Ashley S. Children with fetal alcohol spectrum disorders: Problem behaviors and sensory processing. *American Journal of Occupational Therapy*. 2008;62:265–273.

Greenspan S, Lewis NB. *Building Healthy Minds: The Six Experiences that Create Intelligence and Emotional Growth in Babies and Young Children*. Cambridge, MA: Perseus Books; 1999.

Greenspan S, Weider S. Regulatory disorders. In: Zeanah C Jr, ed. *Handbook of Infant Mental Health*. New York, NY: Guilford Press; 1993;311–325.

Kranowitz CS. *The Out of Sync Child: Recognizing and Coping with Sensory Integration Dysfunction*. New York, NY: Penguin Putnam, Inc; 1998.

Kranowitz CS. *The Out of Sync Child Has Fun: Activities for Kids with Sensory Integration Dysfunction*. New York, NY: Perigee Books; 2003.

Smith K, Gouze K. *The Sensory Sensitive Child: Practical Solutions for Out of Bounds Behavior*. New York, NY: Harper-Collins; 2004.

Wilbarger P. Planning an adequate sensory diet. *Zero To Three*. 1984;1:4–9.

Williams MS, Shellenberger S. *"How Does Your Engine Run?" A Leader's Guide to the Alert Program for Self-regulation*. Albuquerque, NM: Therapy Works Inc; 1996.

Williamson G, Anzalone M. *Sensory Integration and Self-Regulation in Infants and Toddlers: Helping Very Young Children Interact With Their Environment*. Washington, DC: Zero To Three Press; 2001.

TRAUMA

Bryant RA, Mastrodomenico J, Felmingham KL, et al. Treatment of acute stress disorder: a randomized controlled trial. *Archives of General Psychiatry*. 2008;65(5):659–667.

Davidson RJ. Asymmetric brain function, affective style and psychopathology: The role of early experience and plasticity. *Development and Psychopathology*. 1994;6:741–758.

Glaser D. Child abuse and neglect and the brain – a review. *Journal Child Psychology and Psychiatry*. 2000;41:97–116.

Perry BD. The neuroarcheology of childhood maltreatment: The neurodevelopmental costs of adverse childhood events. In: Franey K, Geffner R, Falconer R, eds. *The Cost of Maltreatment: Who pays? We all do*. San Diego, CA: Family Violence and Sexual Assault Institute; 2009:15–37.

Perry BD, Pollard RA, Blakely TL, et al. Childhood trauma, the neurobiology of adaptation and "use dependent" development of the brain: How "states" become "traits." *Infant Mental Health Journal*. 1995;16:271–291.

Strathearn L, Gray PH, O'Callaghan MJ, Wood DO. Childhood neglect and cognitive development in extremely low birth weight infants: A prospective study. *Pediatrics*. 2001;108:142–151.

TREATMENT

American Academy Of Pediatrics. Clinical Practice Guideline: Treatment of the School-Aged Child with Attention-Deficit/Hyperactivity Disorder. *Pediatrics.* 2001;108(4): 1033–1044.

Baradon T, Broughton C, Gibbs I, James J, Joyce A, Woodhead J. *The Practice of Psychoanalytic Parent-Infant Psychotherapy: Claiming the Baby.* London, England: Routledge Publishing Co; 2005

Burns BJ, Hoagwood K, Maultsby LT. Improving Outcomes for Children and Adolescents with Serious Emotional and Behavioral Disorders: Current and Future Directions. In: Epstein MH, Diagnostic Classification Task Force, Stanley Greenspan, M.D., Chair Diagnostic Classification: 0-3: Diagnostic Classification of Mental Health and Developmental Disorders of Infancy and Early Childhood. ZERO TO THREE/National Center for Clinical Infant Programs: Arlington, VA. 1994.

Kutash K, Duchnowski AJ, eds. *Outcomes for Children and Youth with Emotional and Behavioral Disorders and Their Families: Programs and Evaluation Best Practices.* Austin, TX: Pro-Ed; 1998:686–707.

Carmichael-Olson H. Helping individuals with fetal alcohol syndrome and related conditions: A clinician's overview. In: McMahon RJ, Peters RD, eds. *The Effects of Parental Dysfunction on Children.* New York, NY: Kluwer Academic/Plenum Publishers;2002.

Cohen JA, Deblinger E, Mannarino AP, Steer RA. A multi-site, randomized controlled trial for children with sexual abuse-related PTSD symptoms. *Journal of the American Academy of Child and Adolescent Psychiatry.* 2004;43:393–403.

Davis D. *Reaching Out to Children with FAS/FAE.* West Nyack, NY: The Center for Applied Research in Education; 1994.

Hughes, D.A. *Facilitating Developmental Attachment: The Road to Emotional Recovery and Behavioral Change in Foster and Adopted Children.* Northvale, NJ: Jason Aronson Publishing; 2000.

Kinniburgh K, Blaustein M, Spinazzola J, and van der Kolk B. Attachment, self-regulation and competency. *Psychiatric Annals.* 2005;424–430.

Lederman CS, Osofsky JD. Infant mental health interventions in juvenile court: Ameliorating the effects of maltreatment and deprivation. *Psychology, Public Policy, and Law.* 2004;10(1-2):162–177.

Lieberman AF, Silverman R, Pawl JH. Infant-parent psychotherapy. In: Zeanah CH Jr ed. *Handbook of Infant Mental Health.* 2nd ed. New York, NY: Guilford Press; 2000:432.

Masten AS, Bur, K, Coatsworth JD. Competence and psychopathology in development. In: Cicchetti D, Cohen D, eds. *Developmental Psychopathology.* Vol 3, Risk, disorder and psychopathology. 2nd ed. New York, NY: Wiley; 2006.

O'Connor MJ, Kogan N, Findlay R. Prenatal alcohol exposure and attachment behavior in children. *Alcoholism: Clinical and Experimental Research.* 2002;26:1592–1602.

Ponsford J, Willmott C, Rothwell A, et al. Impact of early intervention on outcome after mild traumatic brain injury in children. *Pediatrics*. 2001;108:1297–1303.

Ramsey PG. *Making Friends in School: Promoting Peer Relationships in Early Childhood.* New York, NY: Teacher's College Press; 1991.

Reid R. Self-monitoring for students with learning disabilities: The present, the prospects, the pitfalls. *Journal of Learning Disabilities*. 1996;29:317–331.

Smith T, Groen AD, Wynn JW. Randomized trial of intensive early intervention for children with pervasive developmental disorder. *American Journal of Mental Retardation*. 2000;105:269–285.

Streissguth AP. Fetal Alcohol Syndrome: *A Guide for Families and Communities.* Baltimore, MD: Paul H. Brooks Publishing Co; 1997.

Timmer SG, Urquiza AJ, Zebell NM, McGrath JM. Parent-Child Interaction Therapy: Application to maltreating parent-child dyads. *Child Abuse & Neglect*. 2005;29:825–842.

Wieder S, Greenspan S. The DIR (Developmental, Individual-Difference, Relationship-Based) approach to assessment and intervention planning. *Bulletin ZERO TO THREE: National Center for Infants, Toddlers, and Families*. 2001;21(4):11–19.

Williams MS, Shellenberger S. *How does your engine run? A Leader's Guide to the Alert Program for Self-regulation.* Albuquerque, NM: Therapy Works, Inc; 1996.

Acknowledgments

At this point in a career, the numbers of people to whom I owe a debt of gratitude are many. The clincians at Children's Research Triangle have expanded my knowledge and helped me grow to new ways of understanding children and their relationships. Most especially, Linda Schwartz, Cheryl Pratt, Chrissy Schmidt, Greg Bailey, Erin Telford, Amy Groessl, Anne Wells, and Wendy Messer have challenged and inspired me with their dedication to the children we serve. Sheila Earland manages my time and my calendar; she is my external brain. The families with whom I have worked over the years have given me a realistic picture of their daily lives and have shared their difficulties and hopes with me. They have taught me the importance of giving.

Jeff Link, my exceptional editor, has held the reins tight in taming the overwritten phrase and guiding the flow of each passage and chapter. Maria Fay looked out for my p's and q's and all forms of grammar. Rich McGourty, as my first and foremost reader, has provided honest and frank opinions, always catching the soft spots in the narrative. Bob Rohret, friend extraordinaire, has listened to my laments as I have struggled through difficult sections, always encouraging me with pithy — and, at times, obscene — good humor. Most important, my son Gabe has continued to make sure things run smoothly, freeing me to indulge in writerly pursuits.

And, of course, my wife, Carol, a constant in my life for over forty years who listens patiently and brings me tea while I busily pound away at the keyboard. Last, but far from least, my granddaughters Stav, Noam and Yuval, who make my heart smile with even the thought of them. I am a lucky man.

Index